# Closer to Death: On the Fall of the European Folk Healers

A. Michael Sylm

Published by A. Michael Sylm, 2024.

CLOSER TO DEATH: ON THE FALL OF THE EUROPEAN FOLK HEALERS

**First edition. October 30, 2024.**



ISBN: 979-8227363732

Written by A. Michael Sylm.

Closer to Death:

On the Fall of the European Folk Healers

by A. Michael Sylm

# Introduction

The book will start with our evidence of recreational drug use in the archaeological branch. Then it will move to the concepts of orally transmitted history in culture, followed by pharmaka transmission through writing. I will then talk about the power of belief systems in anthropological context. It will then move to the Greek history of drug use, and on to the rise of christianity.

The witch and the witch trials will be examined and the concepts and historical impacts of private property and the 'hard' analytical sciences will be explored. And then finally, the concept of why the witch crisis is a historical atrocity will be fully noted in the context of drug effects, value, violation, theft, murder, and the misappropriation of wealth will be stated.

# CHAPTER 1: Evidence of Recreational/Cerimonial Drug Use in Prehistory

———

The human story starts in Africa, where the oldest known evidence of a variety of human species occurs. Some of these future astrophysicists migrated north east into the modernly termed Middle East. Some traveled far to the east, some farther north east, but for those making the trek north they reached the edge of the universe: The Scandinavian Ice Sheet.

During the pleistocene period this ice sheet was the borderline, reaching as far south as central Germany, eastwardly to the Russian plains, westward to the Atlantic and northbound to the Arctic. A massive ice sheet, at some areas a mile straight vertical in height with highwinds and subzero temperatures, where mobility may have meant survival.

Many stayed a little closer to more reasonable living situations and stuck around what became known as the Fertile Crescent to include the areas of the Middle East and Southern Europe, and what we are interested in particular is the flora native to those areas. Several species of psychoactive plants are known to have originated or migrated to the area and are still growing there today.

Opium Poppy (*Papaver somniferum*), Mandrake (*Mandragora officinarum*) among many known others, and, as I suspect many of those currently unknown that were once used (or more likely served in combination with substances not known for their psychoactive use) that have been forgotten, overlooked or completely unstudied.

Now it's a little too much in science to assume that people had been using plants for their benefits, sometimes through the roulette of trial and error and for hundreds of thousands of years and acquiring some spoken knowledge of them and their usefulness. Because, well, that would make you and me an ass and the first few chapters of this book useless. But we may have some hard evidence for this. And it was only discovered recently.

In 2024 the scientific journal "Nature" published a study done on Saurian orangutans. While the orangutan was being observed in its natural habitat, one of the observers noticed something, well... different.

The orangutan had a laceration under its eye that was open, quite the gash I might add. It grabbed a leaf of a plant and chewed it–pretty normal stuff, but the orangutan did something amazing shortly after. He began dressing his wound with it.

The orangutan put the chewed up leaf on his open wound. Now this was a plant known by the common name Akar Kuning (*Fibraurea tinctoria*) and happened to be used by natives of the area as an anti-inflammatory, anti-fungal, and antioxidant, a rather potent remedy for wound care. Low and behold the orangutan kept chewing and pasting this until the entire wound was covered and, farther still, for days until the wound was fully healed. Amazing stuff.

So, do primates use medicine? Well, further observations will need to be done in order to rule out chance in this situation which could take a very long time. I mean it's not everyday that an orangutan has a cut that needs attention. But that begs the question, if even orangutans in the wild have a rudimentary form of pharmaka use, when did early humans begin using medicine? What did they use? And when, pray tell, did they start using pharmaka for less obvious reasons such as pain, and quite generally, pleasure?

The Fertile Crescent gave way into what later would be termed the cradle of civilization. There are several pertaining factors that we see emerge from this area: Burials, the first gathering areas and beginnings of settlement, religious ideas and their representations, writing, and eventually pharmacopeias and esoteric manuals.

Burials and elaborate structures abound in the Middle East to include Egypt and Ethiopia. The oldest ever discovered (so far) is the Raqefet Cave Natufian site at Mount Carmel in Israel. This Early Natufian site (approximately 15,000 to 13,700 years ago) is said to be a dramatic shift in human behavior and consciousness. People were beginning to care for their dead, and represent them in some stature beyond the mainstay of their actual lifetimes.

It is in the Raqefet Cave that we see something very sociocultural happening thousands of years ago. Burials and beer (or bread). Symbolism and spiritualism. And, though cross cultural comparisons and major differences in social context may not be the greatest yardstick to measure by, beer in many native cultures is an incredibly important funerary rite in Columbia, even when

Catholicism has come to dominate the natives in the more rural accounts. And that's just one example.

The burial rituals of these individuals would indeed reflect "socio-economic pressures (that) may have coalesced to ignite new symbolic behaviors... Mortuary behavior is one fertile realm for the expression of symbolism and ritual," (Power, Rosen, Nadel). Burial is the easiest place to see culture at work in humans in prehistoric times. It is an indication of people becoming more like we are today.

After analyzing 35 samples at the burial in Raqefet Cave, scientists Power, Rosen and Nadel noted that large and small grass seeds were collected and used, namely wheat and barley. Although the collection of these seeds had always been theorized, the Raqefet Cave seems to present clear evidence of their collection and processing, as well as what may have been a last meal for those buried.

The mortars analyzed had much larger densities of phytoliths (tiny parts of plant insides) than control comparisons which indicated that the carved stones in the cave were used to process, and, possibly, store foods.

So people as long as 13,000 years ago were both burying their dead and processing grains. One benefit of processing grains is the ability to digest them and thus use them to their fullest nutritional potential. If people were improving their health and diet it may have opened up a whole new world of what it meant to be human. One thing is for sure, it would have provided higher survival rates in times of need without the necessity of mass migration during times of drought.

But there is an alternative explanation or, should we say, 'parallel theory' involved with the processed grains at Raqefet Cave: that they weren't making bread, but that they were making beer. To some people this may seem obvious, or at least that they were being made in parallel to one another. But I feel that beer is the much more likely scenario. If for no other reason, it's too easy to make.

We aren't talking frosty glass or ballgame beers here. We are talking about simple beers. In the book "The Shaman's Apprentice" Mark J. Plotkin mentions a staple beer made by the Tukanoan Natives from manioc (*Manihot esculenta*) that they habitually drink. It is simply water, time and you guessed it, human spit– the manioc is literally chewed and spat into the carrying vessel. Boil, and give it time. That's about it.

And you don't even have to spit to make grain based beer, with so many wild yeasts in the air it's almost as if it is supposed to happen. So the suggestion of these containers of remains as being holding tanks, well, if water was added to them for any reason, my friend it will eventually become fermented.

So the argument is something like "Did human civilization start because of bread, or beer?" or put more studiously by Robert J. Braidwood, et al. "Could the discovery that a mash of fermented grain yielded a palatable and nutritious beverage have acted as a greater stimulant toward the experimental selection and breeding of the cereals than the discovery of flour and bread making?" And in my honest opinion it had to be beer, or at least a fermented gruel or porridge.

One of the biggest reasons is that the primitive grain in earlier times would have offered a low return for the labor of those beginning to use them. You just don't have enough material to make bread. Beer is not only self preserving, high in calories, a sociable and thereby a community solidifying drink, and able to send you off to lala land ranting heroic epics, but it is also something that appears naturally in an environment of unideal storage conditions through fermentation. Damp dark storage conditions can even begin malting, or the sprouting of the grain, used as a precursor to more modern brews.

A team of archaeologists led by Li Liu, professor of Chinese archaeology at Stanford University, began considering this in the case of Raqefet Cave. Liu has been an investigator of ancient alcohol consumption practices since her work began in 2015 with Jiajing Wang. What they found at Raqefet Cave in Israel was an ancient style of beer making, after their strict analysis of starches used at the site.

I don't mean to be a buzz kill, but if ancient beer was more like porridge, and the dead at the cave were given a symbolic last meal, and a primitive beer occurs naturally with water, time, and processed grains from the occurrence of wild yeasts in the air, then what is the difference between porridge and beer when food is left to the elements? In this case, malting and brewing.

Interestingly what they discovered was a three-stage brewing process: wheat and barley would be turned into malt by germinating the grain, draining and drying. The dry malt is then crushed and heated. Whalah. Beer. And they recreated this in the laboratory, and get this, the grain afterwards shared a statistically similar shape to those found at the site, a near giveaway that beer was actually used in the funerary rite, not food.

A few thousand years after the Raqefet Cave caveman beers (between 10,000 and 9,000 BC), we see another step in the evolution of culture. Gobekli Tepe was built. The site resides in present day Turkey, and is an outstanding example of early human cultural practices. Megaliths abound at the site, and perhaps just as important socioculturally is the sheer amount of food processing artifacts found there. This was a gathering place, with many 'special' buildings and structures that were interpreted as ritualistic in their function.

And, as the remains of gazelles suggests it was a destination where large scale hunting takes place in the summer and autumn. Some of the artifacts found makes it seem like more of a Grateful Dead concert than an actual hunting gathering. So the natural question is, did they have beer at this party?

In analyzing more than 7000 artifacts at the site, the team of Dietrich, et al. figured that the simple fact that such large scale construction took place, as well as the amount of tools likely used for food and drink production, indicates that large scale workforce feasts took place here. But no permanent settlements as of yet.

Use-wear analysis performed on the grinding equipment indicated the presence of wild barley, wild einkorn, almonds and pistachios. Out of ten types of grinding tools could any one of these specially shaped grinders be for beer specifically? Well, only further investigation will conclude such, but if so it may offer a hint into intoxicants being used by early man for recreational purposes, not just burial rites.

That would mean that people used beer at huge gatherings, that was a *temporary* settlement, before any evidence of permanent settling took place. Perhaps beer and other drugs were enough to stick around for?

Interestingly enough, beers of the more recent past were often more than malt germination, drying, heating, and time. They also added extra oomph. Whether for medicinal or spiritual reasons, or just for kicks, beer was something very different than in our recent history, and was so until the Reformation Period of the Catholic Church. More on this later.

The same archaeological team of Liu and Wang discovered a burial mound site in China with clear evidence of a beer, once again thought to be part of a burial ritual of celebration, commemoration, (or, perhaps, even to become oneself 'close to the experience of death through intoxication,') made from rice (*Orya sp*) Job's tears (*coix lacryma-jobi*) and snake gourd root (*Ageratina altissima*), using a mold starter to kick off the fermentation process. Perhaps these molds, and fungus or even bacterias added to the punch bowl's effects on the mind.

We see some of the first evidence of *drugs* being used either recreationally or spiritually in addition to healing in western Europe around 5900-3500 BC from a study done by Salavert et al. Released in November of 2020. The site seemed to reveal the domestication and early spread through trade (or I suppose taking a souvenir from the Middle East?) of the Opium Poppy.

The study presents some good news and bad news for the researchers: first seeds are easier to find through new sifting techniques used by archaeologists, so botanicals are now commonly searched for at dig sites. The bad news for the researchers is that there is no real way to discern the difference between the opium rich poppy seeds of (*P.somniferum subsp. soniferum L.*) with the opium poor poppy seeds of (*P.somniferum sbsp. Setigerm (DC.) Arcang.*)—the second of which grows wild in the area anyway and does not contain the opium. The modernly cultivated *Subsp. Somniferum L.* is a modern target drug in both health care and on the street and is a very dangerous drug or medicine. The latter, not so much.

Footnote: A friendly reminder: It is also highly addictive. It has recently been tightened on control through sanctions on 28 organizations and people in China over the precursor chemicals used to make the opium derivative Fentynal pain medicine, a street killing drug that has amassed over the counter cures (in some states) of Narcan, a substance that blocks the reception of the drug after lethal amounts are ingested.

Major drug companies are currently under fire and massive fines have been due for their push to prescribe Oxycodone, another derivative of Opium, getting even the elderly addicted to this pain relieving plant. All being said, Morphine itself is a lifesaver during heart attacks and is one of the first medicines administered by First Responders when a patient presents cardiac arrest. More on that later.

An interesting note given by the Salavert, et al. study is that the remains of the currently cultivated Opium poppy are not found (yet) in the neolithic economic trade routes from the Middle East to western Europe or central Europe prior to 5300 bc, but the remains, which leave a definitive difference in signatures when both poppies are compared in burn residues, *have* been determined in charcoal and bone. This may mean that this plant, according to Salavert, "Could be the only crop to have been domesticated in western Europe (by 5900 BCE), given that 50 Early Neolithic sites (5900-4700 cal BCE...) with at least one Opium poppy seed have been recorded through archaeobotanical literature."

And so, since any good science is evidence based we will not assume that people had known about and experimented with herbs and plants in central to northern Europe until the fateful day when a neolithic Einstein was born that decided these plants were a useful cure for pain and can be more than just food. The Einstein I am speaking of is the culprit responsible in 5300 cal BCE of the charred seeds found in structures in central Europe.

It is in these structures that Opium poppy, in my reading of the Salvert et al. study, seemed intentionally used in quantity. And evidence suggests that there was an intense interchange between central Europe and the Mediterranean (the regional origin of Opium poppy) through the appearance of pottery and tool making similarities and intermelding of the two regions.

And the Opium poppy can grow just about anywhere in the world, the more temperate areas of Europe are no exception to its hardiness. At this point, 5300 cal BCE, Opium was well beyond its Mediterranean ecological range, which in some ways indicates that it *was* a commodity at the time. But perhaps a better starting point is not even with the poppy, but instead with native dwelling plants of Europe.

A Bronze age Burial at the cave of Es Carritx in the Balearic Islands (Menorca), off the western coast of Spain provides what could be the first exemplary proof of the consumption of psychoactive substances– not only once mind you, and, not only a particular singular plant species, but several substances– and habitually.

Near 1000 BCE the archipelago of the Baltics was becoming inhabited by humans, and by then they were burying their dead and building megaliths of giant stone structures, dolmens for their dead, and tombs that were cut out of rock. By 1450 BCE however, natural caves were being used to house the dead, blocked off at the entranceway in the same manner a living person's home would be in that area. It was within one of these closed-off natural caves that we met the offender. Uh, or at least what remained of their neatly collected hair that was in an ornamental box at the burial site.

This burial provided a sample of hair that, when exposed to the archaeological tool "Ultra-High-Performance Liquid

Chromatography-High Resolution Mass Spectrometry" (UHPLC-HRMS), scopolamine and atropine alkaloids were detected: tell-tale signs of the scopolamine family of nightshade plants, a plant grouping that includes a slew of psychoactive compounds. Ephedrine was also detected.

The mind bending substances are usually quite elusive to the fossil record and their presence is usually implied in turn by the presence of certain artifacts. One of the most unique parts of this study by Guerra-Doce, et al. is the fact that it was discovered on hair analysis– direct confirmation of consumption in some way.

And the substances were not used once, but over the course of a year. It has proven difficult at many other sites in north and western Europe to find a smoking gun when the nightshades literally grow like weeds in the region, then and now, and are thus easily identified at burials. Yet their *usage* is unconfirmed by the lack of evidence of their ingestion.

The flora that may have been ingested could include some or all of the following: Henbane (*hyoscyamus albus*) and Mandrake (*mondrogora automnalis*), and Joint Pine (*ephedra fragilis*). The use of mandrake or henbane were most probably responsible for the presence of atropine and scopolamine as they grow there in abundance. Joint Pine was most likely the ephedrine, as the pollen had been discovered in a ceramic vessel at a near-by burial site in Son Ferrer, Mallorca– indicating a likely connection to its use and trade.

Once again Opium Poppy (*Papaver somniferum L.*) may have even been used, but its structure has been found to be unstable in archaeobiology as stated above and was thus excluded from this study.

To summarize, the use of pharmaka and psychoactive substances may have an older history than hominids. Some evidence suggests that civilization was established based on the domestication of psychoactive substances that had been in use for millennia prior. Its recreational use and celebratory use, and its function of spiritual intrigue are implied in collective migratory sites and hard evidence from some buried individuals in the Balkans suggests that it was not just used in celebration, but also simply for kicks.

Just a theory but perhaps to some merit. But humans are humans and were humans, people were people. Similar needs, similar wants, similar shortcomings. Maybe nowadays we just have different stuff?

Now in this historical world period, the spiritual world was very much a part of everything that humans said, did, and thought. And eventually wrote about. We cannot even begin to put ourselves there after how far we have removed ourselves from those experiences on the daily. Things like anthropological fieldwork is about as close as we can get, but even then you are on the outside looking in.

And in a way, we don't trust ourselves, our ancestral inheritance, for what they knew, and instead hold life to a standard of proof within a certain margin of error by way of direct evidence, statistical analysis, precision and repeatability. But much is lost in a world of hard science, and was so right from the beginning.

However, there is another way we can travel back in time, and perhaps have some grasp on the mental constructs of the past.

━━━━━━━━

## REFERENCES

Salavert, A., Zazzo, A., Martin, L. *et al.* Direct dating reveals the early history of opium poppy in western Europe. *Sci Rep* 10, 20263 (2020). https://doi.org/10.1038/s41598-020-76924-3

Braidwood, Robert J., Braidwood, Jonathan D. Sauer, Hans Helbaek, Paul C. Mangelsdorf., Cutler, Hugh C., Coon, Carleton S., Lenton, Ralph., Steward, Julian., Oppenheim, Leo A. Did Man Once Live by Beer Alone? (1953). *American Anthropologist, 55.* pp. 515-526.

Baur, Susan Wise. "History of the Ancient World: From the Earliest Accounts to the Fall of Rome." (2001). Amazon Kindle Edition.

Doce, E. Guera,. Herrada, C. Rihuete,. Mico, R., Risch, R., Lull, V., Niemeyer, H. M. Direct Evidence of the Use of Multiple Drugs in Bronze Age Menorca (Western Mediterranean) From Human Hair Analysis.

Laumer, I. B., Rahman, A., Ramaeti, T., Azhari, U., Sri Suci, H., Atmoko, U., Schuppli, C. "Active self-treatment of a facial wound with a biologically active plant by a male Sumatran orangutan." (2024). *Scientific Reports. 14,* 8932.

Liu, Li., Wang, J., Rosenberg, D., Zhao, H., Lengyel, G., Nadel, D. Fermented beverage and food storage in 13,000y-old stone mortars at Raqefet Cave, Israel: Investigating Natufian ritual feasting. (2018). *Journal of Archaeological Science. 21*, 783-793.

Liu, Li., Wang, J., Sun, H., Chen, X. Serving red rice beer to the ancestors ca. 9000 years ago at Xiaohuangshan early Neolithic site in south China. (2023).

Pryor, Francis. "Britain BC: Life in Britain and Ireland Before the Romans." (2003). Amazon Kindle Edition.

Plotkin, Mark J. "Tales of a Shaman's Apprentice: An Ethnobotanist Searches for New Medicines in the Rainforest." (1993). Amazon Kindle Edition.

Jacobs, Andrew., "Tripping in the Bronze Age" 19OCT2023. New York Times. Online edition

Yuval, Noah Harari. "Sapiens a Brief History of Humankind." (2011). Amazon Kindle Edition.

Katz, Josh., Sanger-Katz, Margot., Elleen Sullivan. NYT 05OCT2023 "Some Key Facts About Fentanyl" Online edition.

# CHAPTER 2: Literacy Rates, Problems with Translations, Pharmacopeias and What Makes a Witch

That's where writing comes in. Writing provides some level of concrete proof of practices and compiles years of knowhow. When writing something, especially on clay tablets, there is a cost. Now you may think 'well clay was just lying around.' But the true cost was time. A true cost was who learns to read and write. A true cost was everything you didn't write down. The cost was the hesitation marks. "What do you think we are allowed to forget?" Is a question at cost. And what is worth remembering? What to redact is where power lies.

Written history starts around 2900 BC in what is now Iraq, with clay tablets inscribed with what were basically receipts, or proof of ownership. So by the time of writing, already, we have an incredibly complex society with an active economy, a sense of property, agriculture and animal husbandry. So contrary to our starting point in 'history,' there was a deep past– incredibly deep knowledge of the world had been acquired and survived for thousands of years orally.

At the time writing began, prayers were considered legitimate healing efforts, perhaps as if it were part of a 'doctor's regimen' or treatment. If it seems to work, write it down. And modern anthropologists have noticed that emotional healing is part of a holistic approach to medicine, one in which the entire community can be healed of the fears of impending doom that accompany illness and plague with belief-oriented rituals that changed over time and had invaluable meaning to the tribe's livelihood. Even in the case where a 'witchdoctor's' remedy does not affect the ailment, it has a calming psychological effect through community support, belief systems, and faith, all of which are found important to healing and care.

Mark J. Plotkin, an ethnobotanist, spent a time living and learning from shamans of several villages. His book, and many others like it, places an extreme importance on writing the oral knowledge of a shaman down on paper. This seals the deal on oral knowledge, the transcription will live on long past the lifetime of the individual, existing nearly indefinitely. This transcription, or dare we say "Grimoire" is used as a payment for the shaman's time of teaching, so as to more easily teach future generations. Or, to put it bluntly– corporate greed robbing the weak and poor blindly of their pharmaceutical knowledge.

In a similar vein, David Brusselll of Southern Illinois University did an ethnobotanical field study in the area of Mount Pelion, Greece, where a number of plants and their uses were uncovered by the locals interviewed. Brussell uncovered 225 plants, more than some of them having psychoactive qualities. One recipe of which was adding ivy to wine, known to locals to cause hallucinations.

Brussell makes note of his fieldwork with interesting insight:

*"Having traveled in 71 countries and territories, having gone around the world 4 times, and having done ethnobotanical research in a number of diverse cultures, it has been the author's (Brussell) experience to find that virtually every significant elderly informant consulted has communicated some unique aspect of ethnobotanical data that was singular to that person's own distinct lineage of oral traditions passed down through the ages..." (Every time one of them dies with unrecorded botanical information,) "it is as if a volume of ethnobotanical data goes with them."*

Through Brussell's survey of the Mt Pelion region of Greece, I counted as follows: 4 plants for abortion, 6 plants that served as contraception or aphrodisiacs, 6 narcotics, 1 deadly poison, and 6 non-narcotic plants that do/can cause hallucination depending on amounts ingested. With all of these plants growing wild, an expert herbalist, as a 'witch' would certainly be, could find an entire arsenal of things. And these were threatening to the standard patriarchal society–poisoning royalty, poisoning property owners, land owners, that's serious business. These types of treatments and harms they were often accused of, could be found right under their warts. I mean noses. Or at least certainly in the field close by.

And this type of 'erased' history that Brussell's mentions is well known historically. Oral history and oral pharmacopeias have existed since before traceable history, I mean they must have, and corporations have known this and have poured massive amounts of money into research projects to remote areas in order to locate new 'target drugs' to be used for medicine. The Amazon Rainforest is an incredible example of target drug goldmines as the botanical diversity is unsurpassed.

And not only. The ethnobotanical knowledge known from tribe to tribe due to their presumed seclusion from other societies, brings something entirely unique from tribe to tribe, area to area. Hence, new ideas and new target drugs and medicines are found around every corner. No wonder the corporate lookout, private helicopters and armed escorts for ethnobotanists with Pfizer passcodes.

An interesting thing I would like to point out is that, not only were there different plants in areas, but different languages spoken, and, inevitably different names for the same plants. Even many in terms within the same language. And we see evidence of this in different realms including the Middle East, northern Africa, western Russia and Europe. And even the modern United States and other nations. And unsurprisingly.

A study was done by Dafni, Blanche, Aqil Khatib, et al. for the Journal of Ethnobiology and Ethnomedicine in 2021 documenting different names given to what is now termed Mandrake (*Mandragora autumnalis*), a solanaceae and hallucinogenic plant with a deep past. Their collection was rather phenomenal. From an inventory including Muslim, Turkish, English, German, Dutch and Hungarian languages, "Twenty-eight names in nine languages were connected to various supernatural agents due to their narcotic and hallucinogenic effects," (Dafni, et. al., 2021).

Twenty-eight names for the same plant. Almost all names included a negative connotation of some evil 'negative entity' from 'devil' to 'dragon' to 'goblin' to 'satan' to 'demon.' And those are just the names written down. Did those that were illiterate communicate the same names? Did it vary even farther by region? Town? Or even their uses? It almost certainly did if we were to learn anything from Plotkin and Brussell studies' example.

Although culturally of different origins, early Israeli medico-magical healers, in proper form with shamans and witchdoctors, were using more of these same oral transmissions. According to Gidean Bohak, "the transfer of magical technology seems to have been entirely oral," a fact I suspect is not isolated to the second temple period in Israel. So, the transfer seems not unlike our currently existing shamans in the Amazon Rainforest, or ethnomedical examples in Mt. Pelion, in some respect to sharing oral knowledge and thereby the frailty of retention.

So we get the jist that these concepts and treatments were subject to not only regional deviations, but perhaps even "personal" deviations such as new words for similar (or different) concepts between folk healers. Street names, slang. As stated above, when compared, medico-magical treatments seemed a little like shamanism when it comes to retaining the knowledge therefrom. Though some could write and read, the bulk of the medico-magical work was handled by the have-nots.

To further obscure the past when it comes to words for various psychoactive substances, many Greek words for plants can mean poison *and* cure. Any amount of historical reference in Greek carries this duality and non clarity– if it were to be written down it would have been nearly impossible to distinguish and would depend nearly completely on context (even though they rarely survive in their complete form in papyri, parchment, or paper).

And indistinguishable with good reason. Henbane, Mandrake, Poppies– all contain a cocktail of psychoactive chemicals and other plant compositions that can kill someone if they ingest enough. But it also has useful properties. This ambiguity may have very well played a major, though largely unmentioned, role in the accusations of witchcraft. It was quite the gambit to have this ability with medico-magical tools, a double-edged sword. A position of power for women, and an 'unofficially trained' expert (assassin?) with these capabilities was indeed problematic. And as stated above, directly threatening.

So what do we know? That speaking and referencing plants was diverse even when written in the same language about the exact same thing. And that spoken language varies even more so between region to region, as well as the plants themselves. We know that there were ambiguities between poison and cure. And we also know that there is a powerful historical component to writing when it comes to the erasure and recall of learned medico-magical mainstays. The opposition to those in power were many times erased from history, and the powerful were remembered.

Interestingly enough these elite literary castes of priests did not devise a standard of magico-medical practices in Judaism, it just seems that, if something– anything– worked at least three times, it was fair game to use. Even pagan and foreign deities in Jewish medico-magical remedies, or incantations of demons to be used in exorcisms. Or even calling upon the dead, necromancy, as is seemingly prescribed by scripture in Samuel 28:3-25, when King Saul beacons the Witch of Endor to use her necromancy in order to divinate his future. Or to even kill a witch as was commanded by God "you shall not tolerate a sorceress."

But at the same time there were vivid restrictions on what was considered 'magic.' When the superstitions are removed from this history the difference between the ingroup and the outgroup, really seems to be literacy. The actual study of such literary attempts left behind after the slow process of trial and error were the basis of what became a rudimentary type of healing and wound care for the early Israelites, and presumably most other regions.

So there is a strange connection here: sometimes it's ok to use 'the devil's' plants. Sometimes when learned practitioners could not work their 'medico-magical' knowhow they resorted to witch healers that used certain 'other or unlearned' substances and techniques to heal. And we still see some of these psychoactive medico-magical remedies used today with the occurrence of nightshade plants, one chemical derivative namely, that is a crucial med in every ER doctor's crash cart: Atropine.

As stated above, the practices were something more 'medico-magical' then what we think of today as 'medicine.' Some of these procedures seem today to be verging on the absurd. One example, and there are many others, is a piece of that history from around the period of the rise of Christianity, dating as far back as 200 BC in compiled documents such as the Greek Magical Papyri, which was a collection of writings from 200 BC to around 400 AD.

One of these 'devilish' nightshade plants, Henbane (*Hyoscyamus niger*), was used and recorded in the writings from the sixth century by Alexander of Tralles. Being pestered by royalty, as many great medico-magical practitioners were, he was constantly asked to replace his 'methodic' treatments (which were the more modern medical treatments) with the 'natural' remedies (which were the ones we would now call magical recipes). Oddly enough this magical recipe called for the use of Henbane as the substance known (to some medico-magical technicians) to heal gout.

Included in this recipe are some seemingly 'magical' ideas on how to uproot this plant. Reading this today you may be thinking more along the lines that it was laid out in such a way in order to treat the plant with utmost care and respect. Why? Today we would know that the act of getting the juice of the root itself on the hand would have quite unknowable effects on the body as the topical absorption route can still be fatal or hallucinogenic, especially in high concentrations– you don't even have to necessarily touch your eye or mouth to the crushed plant.

When placed in combination with other plants, the absorption could be even more deadly or delirium inducing, whether the plant is seemingly psychoactive or not– even some of the most mundane seeming things could also easily be a catalyst, such as some of the plants stated above in Brussell's survey. Psychoactive plants are not something to take lightly, and if you were in the plant retriever's shoes you'd probably determine that you were possessed by the spirit of the plant, evil or satan if exposed to the juices. Given your time and place in history– you're bewitched.

Therefore, the act of pulling the plant was quite the process even if the reasoning was off, they went to incredible lengths to avoid mishandling it. It's not like they had latex gloves or something. The words of Alexander of Tralles:

*"Dig around the holy plant, that is henbane, when the moon is in Aquarius or Pisces, before sunset, without touching the root. Dig with these two fingers of the left hand – the thumb and the fore-finger – and say: "I tell you, I tell you, holy plant, tomorrow I will call you to the house of NN... (and) I adjure you by the great name Iaoth Saba ^ oth, the god who founded the earth and stopped the sea in spite of the influx of rising rivers, he who dried up Lot's wife and made her salty. Take the spirit of your mother Earth, and her power, and dry up the rheumatic flux of the feet or the hands of this man or that woman." On the next day, before sunrise, take the bone of any dead creature, dig it (the henbane root) up with this bone, take the root and say: "I adjure you by the holy names Iaoth, Saba ^ oth, Ad ^ onai, El ^ oi." And as you take it, throw on the root some salt and say: "Just like this salt will not grow, let not the illness of this man or that woman (grow)." Then take the tip of the root and tie it around the patient as an amulet – but make sure it does not get wet – and hang the rest (of the root) above the hearth for 360 days."*

Waiting a day to dig it up would allow the outside of the exposed root to dry and weep out its poisons. Even harden the skin surrounding it. To throw salt on it would be to further draw out (only) water and concentrate the root. To only use the tip of the root as an amulet, is providing a small topical dose to the patient.

Mandrake retrieval legends are even more outlandish. Going as far as saying similar time and place necessities and the need for a dog to drag out the root by attaching its leash to it very carefully. The next step was to cover your ears, place food a distance from the dog, and when the root comes out it screams and well, the dog dies, and there's your plant.

But if it worked, it was undeniable as a treatment– even if it was of 'the devil' or stigmatized with a similar evil entity when it came to the beginnings of medico-magical formulae. Many years later, the elites will switch paths (though not completely) and looking back into the books they wrote over the years this 'whatever works' method would no longer be the case. In what would later be determined a 'witch' legally would be mandated by the Catholic Church and take many years to refine to hysteria, many years of redaction, and many years of immeasurable destruction of culture that further led to the Inquisitions and mass colonial murder.

---

## REFERENCES

Bohak, Gideon. A History of Jewish Magic. Amazon Kindle Edition. (2008).

Brown, Peter J. *Understanding and Applying Medical Anthropology* (1998) Mayfield Publishing Company.

Brusselll, David Eric. Medicinal plants of Mt. Pelion, Greece. *Economic Botany*. 58.

Dafni, Amots., Blanche, C., Khatib, S.A., Petanidou,T., Aytac, B., Pacini, E., Kohazorva, E., Geva-Kleinberger, A., Shahvar, S., Dajic, Z., Klug, H.W., Benitez, G. In search of traces of the mandrake myth: the historical, and ethnobotanical roots of its vernacular names. (2021). *Journal of Ethnobiology and Ethnomedicine. 17*(68).

Maravi, P., Atropine eye-drop-induced acute delirium: a case report. 2020 National Institutes of Health (NIH) (.gov) https://www.ncbi.nlm.gov article PMC7223267

Plotkin, Mark J. (1993). The Shaman's Apprentice (Kindle ed.). Amazon.

Wade, Nicholas.,"Scanning an Ancient Biblical Text That Humans Fear to Open" NYT 05JAN2018 Online edition

Berlin, A., Brettler, M.Z. (2003). The Jewish Study Bible (Kindle ed.). Amazon.

# CHAPTER 3: Bacchic Mysteries and the Pagan Continuity Hypothesis

The Bacchic Mysteries were festival-type rituals held throughout the Roman empire starting around 200 BC running well into the Imperial Era of Rome (ending around the time the empire was split, roughly 395 AD, also around the time the new testament to the holy bible was written). There were large, chaotic public events in the name of Bacchus, an admired deity, the showcase of which was a highly preferred and potent wine infusion of hallucinogenic quality made with a secret recipe: most likely ivy and some other types of herbs that remain a mystery. What we see here through the use of potent wine and the flare of a private venue for participation is something of a trade off between preferred deities.

To some it may be presumed obvious that Christianity was a continuation of many pagan tendencies. A kind of amalgamation of Judiasim and Paganism as well as Gnosticism. But some may not be so easily convinced. I'll let you as a reader look into the deity similarities of Jesus and Bacchus on your own, but I'll lay out some of the connections relevant to this discussion.

The Bacchic Mysteries were a popular festival that promised its initiates a wonderful life in the here and now and ever after. The rites included the drinking of wine, as the associated deity Bacchus (Dionysus) was the god of wine. He was also, however, the god of Frenzies, and in this way bore some resemblance to Pan (the namesake of 'Panic' mind you) with outcomes of discordance and chaos.

These Bacchic rites were not for the faint of heart, and they were intense, intoxicating, uplifting, and nightmarish in many ways. Animals would be thrown to the crowd of initiates, torn to pieces and eaten raw, while the music raged in cacophony and the initiates danced and trampled in the blood. This was the type of thing meant to be therapeutic, life changing.

Rome had a nac for recognizing the darker urges of man, and in the rites tried to purge those feelings so as to make more upright citizens in a process termed 'catharsis,' a similar type of letting of emotion was done through theater. But the Bacchic Rites were not the type of thing you could walk away from unscorned, untraumatized, with many strong emotions. Happy to be home afterwards.

The wine, as pointed out in the Brussell Survey most likely contained Ivy, a vine known to the locals even today to be hallucinogenic in high quantities. It most likely contained other ingredients as well. Wine, just like beer, had more of a kick to it in the past and was meant to take your head in all kinds of directions, to bring you a step closer to death.

After hundreds of years of these behaviors, it seems, and this is just my own vague assumption, when Rome's days of conquest began to wane, Gnosticism came knocking as well as a rudimentary Catholicism. Peter The Apostle of Christ had arrived in Rome and began spreading the gospel of Jesus. However, his testament to Christ was yet to be written.

And as is practically needless to point out, Christianity has, and still does, adapt to other cultures; only these days, instead of the big man Christ they are having to adapt, it's lesser Saints to the Catholic order. This can be seen in nearly every Latin American country, and even closer looks at regions will show this overt behavior to adapt the Gospel to the needs of the community it is projected upon.

In "Magical Writing in Salasaca" Peter Wogan states: "San (Saint) Gonzalo's healing only occurs in the negative sense of canceling out his own lethal attacks; he is distinctly unlike other Catholic saints who increase fertility or bring good luck, and his prices are exorbitant." This saint has a witchy-type black magic to kill if a person's name is taken off of a baptism record. Members of this Ecuadorian tribe have to pay a black magic practitioner to fix the situation. This may seem odd to some, but does not seem to be a rarity in central and south america to my knowledge.

Or elsewhere. There are many saints in the Catholic Order, and you pray to them for specific reasons. Good luck, family issues, drug use—all different saints to pray to.

That being stated, Peter, that same apostle that lived in Rome shortly after Christ's crucifixion, has the only Testament to mention both the Eucharist, and the water to wine miracle, accredited to himself. So bear that in mind when it is said that through the Testament of Peter, Christ became more like Bacchus, the most popular deity at the time in Rome, with the most festivities, also curiously, around the time the Bacchic Rites stopped popping up.

In this hypothesis, Christianity was like a diet, zero cal, caffeine-free version of the Bacchic rites. The theology can almost be seen basically like a sales pitch: you don't need to sacrifice animals anymore because Christ was sacrifice enough for the rest of eternity, you will still have a good afterlife, you still will have a good life, we'll even come right to your door, and get this... you can make the sacred wine in your own homes. Joining new cults as initiates and experiencing secretive rites was all the rage. Everyone's favorite flavor was Bacchus, so why not make it even better?

What the Bacchus cult accomplished with frenzies, to the first Christians (and modern people agree I'm sure) was shameful. I can't speak for those involved, but I imagine that most of the people didn't enjoy being traumatized over and over again by acute losses of complete control. Though it may be that the draw was a little more to the intoxication than anything else. Perhaps it was a 'stylized poppy' as Brussell suggested. Making religion a literal 'opiate of the masses' to quote Marx.

And many towns had their own rites for their local favorite deity. The secretive process of becoming an initiate basically allowed you access to various forms of designer drugs as they would be called today. And you must recall that plants interact differently when working in parallel with other plants. That's just organic chemistry 101.

As an example, the South American tribal brew Ayahuasca is case and point. It is a mixture of these two species: (*Psychotria viridis*) leaves, and the (*Banisteriopsis caapi*) vine. The first and most psychoactive of the two plants doesn't do much without the other plant, a generally useless plant mind you, that just so happens to be a Monoamine Oxidase Inhibitor (MAOI). When the two are mixed, look out for giant boa constrictor gods

And with all this madness, in luck for christianity, Rome was ready to move on. According to Yulia Ustinova: "Bacchic mania might at times be regarded as excessive, therefore in need of some state control." And this wine, if it contained a sizable amount of Ivy, enough to hallucinate making a little is making a lot. And as it sounds, incredibly easy.

And even though the first Christians may have done this at home, you should not.

State control was needed, but it seems that the Christians held the answer–not only to better control the festive ritualistic cults that abounded, but also to unite the vast area of the empire under one religious loom that would later define Rome, and survive to this day through the Vatican CIty.

Bacchus and Christ share many similarities, and it is not hard to see how the Eucharist could have been a tamer version to the Bacchic rites, even with all intoxicants to boot. Now there is no certainty in this, but who knows. What we do see, rather clearly, is a scenario where mass ceremonial public intoxication moved to a private setting, permitting the Bacchic right alternative to a more concrete and controlled environment. And we know the drugs were there, assuming Muraresku is correct in his analyses of artwork found in the 'lesser seen' areas of the Vatican, where ivy and grapes are painted everywhere and where women played a once greater role in the roots of Roman Christianity as they once did in the Bacchic Rites as the wine bearers. Women being so involved in the cult of Christ was certainly a Gnostic objective, not necessarily a Catholic one.

But the Eucharist was to serve a purpose, and the mainstay of becoming 'close to god' or presumably 'closer to death.' And it was just these designer drug efforts that liberated the initiates from their troubles with the fickleness of life in general. According to Ustinova: "the encounter with the divine was perceived as mingling with the god, and this temporal unity with the divine was the aim of the initiation." The rites at the time were considered both a 'possession' by the deity and so it would very well follow that, through transmogrification of bread and wine into the body and blood of Jesus, to consume the Eucharist was to become closer with God by way of direct bodily consumption and being possessed by Christ. The aim was indeed to become closer to God. Now as far as I know the Eucharist isn't like this anymore (although there is a brand of wine considered sacramental wine, that only the church knows the ingredients to), but it most certainly had to be in order to compete with the other cults in Rome at the time.

So to summarize what we have seen: The desire of intoxication and medical treatment helped drive the care and domestication of plants. Plants that were dangerous were given deep lore for their possible need to be handled with care, and were used by those learned and unlearned individuals in a sort of trade off of what worked (trial and error). Things that worked were repeated, but loosely organized in language of the craft, where the learned wrote, the unlearned held in mind and orally–making for an array of vocabulary even when referring to the same plants within the same area of the world. With diverse language and unwritten knowhow, the witch was easily made into a target in society, but until the height of witch hysteria were acceptable teachers and practitioners.

The line between poison and cure was not clear, and with good reason, most of the psycho/somatically active plants were indeed, incredibly dangerous. Mixing chemicals could have serious consequences. Some of these intoxicants were used in public ceremonial outcroppings later to be moved to more private tamer settings (as seen in more modern psychedelic and meditative scenarios) by the influx of Christianity's adaptation to the Western Philosophies and adapting to Roman cultic practices and cultural influence. A badly mixed batch was poison in its concentration, and got one a little too close to death.

And we see this adaptation over and over again throughout the history of the Catholic Church. Kind of this 'adding' to theology things that are influencing it in order to stay ahead of the other cults. And the takeover wasn't always peaceful either. Actually, it never was. Christians were known to burn down buildings, smash up temples and statues, deface property, and burn books as in Acts 19:19-20 that describes a mass magical book burning once Paul exorcised a demon. Interestingly, Acts 19:20 says this has a value, perhaps a harking battle cry to commandeer grimoires in the open war on Satan and exploit the European folk-healing lot as this essay is suggesting. Yet, somehow the

Christians got ahold of the secret Bacchus recipe, or an improvement of it, and they sort of bought up the other cults of Rome.

---

REFERENCES


DeKorne, J. (2011). Psychedelic Shamanism: The Cultivation, Preparation, and Shamanic Use of PsychoTropic Plants (Kindle ed.). Amazon.

Brusselll, D. E. (2004). Medicinal Plants of Mt. Pelion, Greece. *Economic Botany*, *58*, S174–S202. http://www.jstor.org/stable/4256917

Wogan, P. (2003). Magical Writing in Salasaca: Literacy and Power in Highland Ecuador (Kindle ed.). Amazon.

Muraresku, B.C. (2020). Immortality key: the secret history of the religion with no name (Kindle ed.). Amazon.

Ustinova, Y. (2017) Divine mania: alteration of consciousness in ancient Greece (Kindle ed.). Amazon.

Nixey, C. (2017). The Darkening age: the christian destruction of the classical world (Kindle ed.). Amazon.

# CHAPTER 4: The Rise of Christianity and the Destruction of Folk Healing in Europe

A pivotal moment in the history of the Church was when Emperor Constantine of Rome converted to Christianity (unwillingly as I've heard) in 337 AD moments before he died. This opened the floodgates for what became a well established religion in Rome that persists to this day.

Christianity seemed to be part of the answer to civil unrest and cultural irregularities that resorted from Rome stretching its boundaries across large swaths of land. Before its widespread approval, there was nothing that seemed to make people feel united, not even a common currency.

The quest that concerned 'uniting' the Roman people would not be a pretty or peaceful one. The Church, through a series of theological documents written by clergy that were later nearly deified as saints declared open war on the forces of 'evil' which would come to include simply any religious facet that did not encumber the weight of the (catholic brand) cross.

This was a slow and meticulous process, but one that would come to include many crusades, inquisitions, and a formula used to aid in conquests of foreign lands during colonialism– the resulting violence of the church literally had no boundary.

And neither did their hold on medico-magical practices, designer drug alcohols and military force. When it came to medico-magical practices, the church was beginning to design the right way and the wrong way of doing things in their open war against satan, i.e. describing the witch as a legal entity, establishing Hospitalar units within its ranks as well as running one of the first hospital systems in 1099–the Hospital of Saint Lazarus in Jerusalem. Assuredly using the latest technologies available, this hospital was for christians that made the trek on pilgrimage to Israel as well as a treatment center for many of those afflicted with leprosy.

By the time the Church had debated what was heretical, the Albigensian Crusade took place against the Cathars whose teachings were deeply Gnostic in nature, but, of course, one that did not deny the belief in Christ. The Cathars were legally defined as 'heretics' by the Church, a word that would be used to describe the outgroups, and be the staple of many witch trials to come. By some estimates one million people died in the Albigensian Crusade's 20 year genocide in southern France from 1209-1229. And that was only the first of many.

As far as designer drug alcohols, the Church maintained a hold on breweries and the contents thereof, wine vineyards and their contents and the distribution, protected by military enforced trade routes. With thousands of brewing monasteries and the first brewery in Europe, Catholic monks made many advances on brewing technologies. Indeed, the Church defined what beer was made out of, a very important device of near corporate power, and eventually maintained a monopoly on gruit (herbs and plants used in beers to preserve, flavor and add umph) stupefying an entire region with whatever they pleased.

When it came to military prowess, the Church had several personal military sects to include the Templar Knights, and during the First Crusade to take back Jerusalem for Rome, even gave the citizens an ultimatum that was, in simple words, a trap—citizens had to pay their way to be in the military, to include food, and fight for God regardless of their participation in the military or not—those that fought got a free ride to Heaven, those who didn't were ostracized by their communities as cowards and sinners, and, well, broke and indebted to the Church.

The witches were just one outgroup the church had in their sights for destruction. For the purposes of this discussion one of the first documents that pertained to witches was the 'Canon Episcopi' which was believed to be originally composed in 906 AD, the manuscript first described witchcraft as a crime that should be punished. It is uncertain by the time of its authorship what exactly made someone a witch, but the inclusion of the phrase: "Thoroughly eradicate the pernicious art of divination and magic, invented by the devil, from their parishes" says a bit of a mouthful. After all, elite and freelance medico-magical practitioners alike used mandrake for example.

The Holy Bible, which is considered the laws and word of God, (and thereby the ultimate law although not the same as what is 'legal' at this time in Rome) makes several mentions of the witches and even allows their consultation, even though God commanded not to tolerate a sorceress, making things like heresy and witchcraft difficult to define. Naturally, at the time of the Canon Episcopi's writing, punishments for witchcraft were not doled out nearly as often as what was to come. But the concepts still remain as mentioned by the Episcopi: that witchcraft was the invention of Satan, that witchcraft was an illusion beset by the Devil and demons, and that it should be removed... all to be repeated and refined for a thousand years to increasing intensity.

It was not until the Renaissance and the Reformation period of the Church that we see witchcraft as a crime reach extremes in prosecutions. The accusations however, did not seem to have a stable foundation in logic even for this time. The powers that were associated with the witch: flying, transformation, weather control, etc., were considered an illusion–but only to the witch! The Church is still far from accepting the existence and prevalence of magic as impossible. What the Church was actually emphasizing is that the acts of the witch are simply powerful illusions contrived by the Devil, to trick *the witch themselves* into thinking they have the power of demons–and interestingly this whole scenario is a punishment by God for sinning and turning to demons for assistance in some task. Furthermore, it was God himself that commanded these demons to punish the affected individual/s for sin and noncompliance, striking them with drought and hail. Anything to sell gruit laced beer I presume.

Courts of the middle ages make several mentions of cases that *were revised after their documentation* to fit a mold that became increasingly stereotypical. These have-nots were considered with the same out-group descriptions as, ironically, even the christians were in the past. Witches were accused of many things that were simply impossible. Witches under torture were accused of being immune to pain by way of help from demons–as if some show of strength, dignity or innocence were impossible for those accused. Witches pregnant with a married man's child would be persecuted–not for men cheating on their wives with them–but for the witch sending a demon to steal a man's semen while he was sleeping and insert it into herself. All around appalling circumstances to say the least. To think that a 'witch' (or should we say 'a woman with strength and expertise'?) could get a rich man to fall in love with her, get her pregnant, or die by her herbs was simply too much to bear.

More realistically the witches were using gruit illegally. Abortions, poisons, cures, aphrodisiacs, fertility help, lactation help, getting high, pain relief–these were all things that these medico-magical practitioners were able to do. Not only were times changing to place a value on this information but the fact that it was the 'lesser sex' with these types of threatening capabilities made them something the Church would feel the need to eradicate. Eye witnesses during the Reformation periods of the Church raised arguments, just as the pure onslaught that science was beginning to prove, was that these individuals, that claimed to have these powers, were sound asleep while these things were taking place.

Some sporadic arguments during this time period repeated that there was an ointment, or in some cases a drink of some kind that was taken or put across the skin or orifice and that the witch fell into a deep sleep, waking up and believing that they had done these fantastic things. And it was incredibly believable. To the 'witch.' Psychologically you have someone having vivid and lucid dreams. As mentioned before, these dreams seem to run in a similar vein, perhaps like a shamanistic 'plant teacher.' Anyone who has ever taken too much Dramamine for motion sickness on a plane could probably contest to the ease of belief from these soporific induced lucid dreams. My experience was asking the stewardess for some more of that incredible ice cream. They didn't give us ice cream, nor did they ever offer. Except I suppose I really was kind of flying right? Perhaps I'm a witch then.

You also have a time period of magical thinking, and of course there are outstanding coincidences such as the occasional occurring famine. Furthermore, there are those with cruel intent, purposeful and wrongful acts such as sneaking into the neighbors' home at night and souring all their milk chemically. All of this could and would make someone themselves feel rather powerful, and feared as well.

So superstitions aside, what we have here is a powerful herbalist with deep knowledge of hallucinogens, poisons, healing remedies and several areas that empower women specifically when it comes to child bearing (abortion and aphrodisiacs). As much as the church wanted the witches to hold no power without God, they actually kind of did. They could play God just as well as any other doctor. The difference is that sometimes, their intention was to harm, something deemed unethical even by the standards of doctoring in the renaissance.

And what exactly were the drugs that made this whole fiasco believable to the witch? The soporific drugs alluded to by eye witness skeptics were most likely those drugs with the most lore as they were hardy plants growing across the entirety of Europe, and even into the Middle East. Undoubtedly there were others, but the ones with the most lore are very likely candidates because of their widespreadness and simplicity in identification.

Deadly nightshade is one of these plants. Believe it or not it is labeled one of the World Health Organization's target plants for its production of chemicals that can be reduced and purified into Atropine. Atropine as mentioned earlier is an essential drug in emergency medicine in the case of ventricular fibrillation, and even is used in the military as an antidote to chemical attack. There are factories where these plants are 'milked' in a process that aspirates the chemicals from its roots. It is known to cause hallucinations in many people, and is used as a recreational drug in some areas of the world. And this plant grows all over the place, native to Europe, but has since spread with global trade. Too much will make you sleep. Well, something more like a 2-3 day coma.

Henbane (Datura stramonium) is another one of these easily identified substances that grows not only just about everywhere, but is also found in fields of crops. Also known as Jimson Weed it is the culprit in the famous Jamestown mass hallucination scenario, and is a deadly poison in high quantities. Henbane is used to this day in America, namely the western and southwestern states as a cheap high and goes by many street names. Yep, put you in a coma.

Mandrake is native to the middle east but has since spread. It had been contested for many thousands of years to contain aphrodisiac, anesthetic and hallucinatory properties. There was once an illegal trade of mandrake that involved counterfeit mandrake charms for people to wear. They were simply anatomical trinkets sold for big bucks on the market as authentic mandrake charms. Mandrake is legendary and is mentioned in the Bible, making it a popular medico-magical go-to.

In the realm of suspicion and superstitions were also real life happenings and reasons for such paranoia. According to Kohnen-Johannsen and Kayser, "In addition to hallucinogenic and analgesic effects, nightshades have a history of being used as poisons, for example, a wave of unexplainable mortality in the French high-society was attributed to these plants." Most likely these poisonings led to witch prosecutions.

All of these plants are associated with witchcraft, and many of them are also associated with healthcare. And we can be certain there are thousands of others. So what it seems to me, is that there was a vague timeline of things that occurred–

The witch stereotype was most developed within the publications of "The Ant Hill" (1447) and "The Hammer of Witches," (1486). William IV, Duke of Bavaria, passed the Reinheitsgebot in 1516, which restricted beer ingredients to water, barley, and hops, ending the Church's stronghold on beer additives at least in Germany. Martin Luther was beginning to shake up the Catholic domination of Western religion (1517). Germany interestingly enough had one of the highest rates of incinerating drug-using witches. The church, with seemingly no more control over the designer drug market of the region may have had it out for the have-not orally trained faith healing 'sorceress.'

The Microscope was invented in 1590 upending much of what was once thought about disease and a concept called 'spontaneous generation' of things like maggots and other animals–alchemy was beginning to break apart into rudimentary forms of the hard sciences and iatrochemical medicine was beginning to overtake the medicinal use of plants. Newton invented calculus in the 1660s, and developed laws that can determine the physical world and worlds around us. In 1690, John Locke had written his treatise on the value and ownership of private property. And in this 100 years the church had to definitely be looking for new avenues on how to make a profit for itself. Inquiring of the witches' motives and uses of herbal knowledge by now had an obvious value. To burn the witch and the grimoire, or the 'oral grimoire,' by now was lucrative business.

Charles Darwin wrote "Origin of Species" 1859 upending the Church's very own creation story–ironically, it was a Monk, Geogor Mendel that provided the missing link to complete Charles Darwin's theory of evolution in 1866– finding experimental proof of dominate and recessive traits, a rudimentary form of genetics.

What it seems to me, through this sequence of events, is that the Church's hold on designer-drug beers was slipping and the Church's view was changing about their knowledge of gruit. To persecute those who used the sort of 'gruit' substances illicitly, were using something the church saw value in. And a new market was opening up–the hard sciences. Plants were being reduced to bare chemicals, the folk healers, with a little help of stereotyping and demonizing were now a wealth of botanical knowledge that could be used for profit, exploitation and 'learned' medicine.

The havenots were ridiculed, tortured, interrogated, tried and burned, along with their historical knowhow... or were they? Who's to say these oral pharmacopeias by the time of refined alchemies weren't written somewhere to be lost in a sea of words that are as unique to the area as they were to the witch? And they had no protection from it. They were easy targets. Confiscation of grimoires, the banning of books, the burning of books (i'm assuming keeping a copy for the Church's secret library first) and burning the oral craft out of existence through the trials, protected the Church from what may have been their saving investment– botanical knowledge in a world beginning to look for medicine.

You have to remember that throughout a thousand and more years, the Church was a cash cow–mandatory tithes, taxes, confiscated gold from conquests, even selling relics to wealthy elite and kings, the Church was a major influence, and as the paradigm began to shift they must have noticed and found new avenues of investment. The witch trials were just another exploitation. They doubled down on superstitions and the Church's mission while having the changing paradigm in mind– that these plants may have not been of the devil but were definitely doing something to people. Mandrake is one of those long running examples–long used in medicine, medico-magical remedies, and abused by 'witches,' and of course, of Biblical popularity.

Is this a crackpot theory? I'm sure many would think so. But the fact of the matter is that the church ran since day one an exploitation racket, and these exploitations still exist to this day in the rainforests of Africa and South America. New target drugs, new recipes for various ailment treatments are a huge industry. Pharmaceuticals are a major point of investment for many major market players and, well, make the world a better place. To treat the folk healers of Europe much in the way of modern drug users in the war on drugs, aside from the burning, is a huge market as well.

For many years prisons were filled to capacity with non-violent drug offenders. Recently many states in America have relaxed laws on marijuana to the discontent of the federal government, building tax revenue for those states, tourism–a brand new industry for some of the hard core advocates and those who took up the offer of start-up incentives in the early days of the laws changing.

The formula for persecution and exploitation of drug users never really changed all that much in the fact that it was centered on profit potential. Anything from acquiring new slang to supplying the drug dealers has (and had) been used. To project current and recent history onto the past is a long shot, but only at most. As stated before, people are people and have always been with similar wants, needs and desires, similar bewilderments and similar problems.

## REFERENCES

Peters, E., Kors, A.C. Witchcraft in Europe, 400-1700: A Documentary History. (2000). University of Pennsylvania Press

Russell, J.B. Witchcraft in the Middle Ages. (1984). Cornell University Press.

Bauer, SW. (2013). The History of the Renaissance World: From the Rediscovery of Aristotle to the Conquest of Constantinople (Kindle ed.). Amazon.

Bauer, SW. (2010). The History of the Medieval World: From the Conversion of Constantine to the First Crusade (Kindle ed.). Amazon.

Jones, D. (2017). The Templars: The Rise and Spectacular Fall of God's Holy Warriors (Kindle ed.). Amazon.

Riley-Smith, J. (1987) The Crusades: A History (Kindle ed.). Amazon.

Hatsis, T. (17AUG2015). The Witches Ointment: The Secret History of Psychedelic Magic ( Kindle ed.). Amazon.

Thomas, C. (2006). Confusion, agitation, and severe hallucination in a teenager: the boy's friends reported that earlier that night, he had been seen smoking marijuana and drinking herbal tea. Clinical Advisor, 9(9). https://go.gale.com/ps/i.do?p=AONE&u=uphoenix&id=GALE|A153292766&v=2.1&it[1]

Mutebi RR, Ario AR, Nabatanzi M, Kyamwine IB, Wibabara Y, Muwereza P, Eurien D, Kwesiga B, Bulage L, Kabwama SN, Kadobera D, Henderson A, Callahan JH, Croley TR, Knolhoff AM, Mangrum JB, Handy SM, McFarland MA, Sam JLF, Harris JR, Zhu BP. Large outbreak of Jimsonweed (Datura stramonium) poisoning due to consumption of contaminated

---

1. https://go.gale.com/ps/i.do?p=AONE&u=uphoenix&id=GALE%7CA153292766&v=2.1&it=r&sid=ebsco

humanitarian relief food: Uganda, March-April 2019. BMC Public Health. 2022 Mar 30;22(1):623. doi: 10.1186/s12889-022-12854-1. PMID: 35354446; PMCID: PMC8969350.

Sara, A. Review on Pharmacology of Atropine, Clinical Use and Toxicity. Biomedical and Pharmacology Journal, 15(2) June 2022. DOI: http://dx.doi.org/10.13005/bpj/2408

Kohnen-Johannsen, K.L., Kayser, O. Tropane Alkaloids: Chemistry, Pharmacology, Biosynthesis and Production. Molecules. 2019 Feb; 24(4): 796. doi: 10.3390/molecules24040796 PMCID: PMC6412926 PMID: 30813289

Alizadeh A, Moshiri M, Alizadeh J, Balali-Mood M. Black henbane and its toxicity - a descriptive review. Avicenna J Phytomed. 2014 Sep;4(5):297-311. PMID: 25386392; PMCID: PMC4224707.

Arbia F, Ayari-Gribaa O, Souilem F, Chiboub W, Zardi-Berguaoui A, Jannet HB, Ascrizzi R, Flamini G, Harzallah-Skhiri F. Profiles of the Essential Oils and Headspace Analysis of Volatiles from Mandragora autumnalis Growing Wild in Tunisia. Chem Biodivers. 2019 Oct;16(10):e1900345. doi: 10.1002/cbdv.201900345. Epub 2019 Sep 11. PMID: 31390142.

Srinivasan P, Smolke CD. Biosynthesis of medicinal tropane alkaloids in yeast. Nature. 2020 Sep;585(7826):614-619. doi: 10.1038/s41586-020-2650-9. Epub 2020 Sep 2. PMID: 32879484; PMCID: PMC7529995.

## BIBLIOGRAPHY

Peters, E., Kors, A.C. Witchcraft in Europe, 400-1700: A Documentary History. (2000). University of Pennsylvania Press

Russell, J.B. Witchcraft in the Middle Ages. (1984). Cornell University Press.

Bauer, SW. (2013). The History of the Renaissance World: From the Rediscovery of Aristotle to the Conquest of Constantinople (Kindle ed.). Amazon.

Bauer, SW. (2010). The History of the Medieval World: From the Conversion of Constantine to the First Crusade (Kindle ed.). Amazon.

Jones, D. (2017). The Templars: The Rise and Spectacular Fall of God's Holy Warriors (Kindle ed.). Amazon.

Riley-Smith, J. (1987) The Crusades: A History (Kindle ed.). Amazon.

Hatsis, T. (17AUG2015). The Witches Ointment: The Secret History of Psychedelic Magic ( Kindle ed.). Amazon.

Thomas, C. (2006). Confusion, agitation, and severe hallucination in a teenager: the boy's friends reported that earlier that night, he had been seen smoking marijuana and drinking herbal tea. Clinical Advisor, 9(9). https://go.gale.com/ps/

i.do?p=AONE&u=uphoenix&id=GALE|A153292766&v=2.1&it=r&
2

Mutebi RR, Ario AR, Nabatanzi M, Kyamwine IB, Wibabara Y, Muwereza P, Eurien D, Kwesiga B, Bulage L, Kabwama SN, Kadobera D, Henderson A, Callahan JH, Croley TR, Knolhoff AM, Mangrum JB, Handy SM, McFarland MA, Sam JLF, Harris JR, Zhu BP. Large outbreak of Jimsonweed (Datura stramonium) poisoning due to consumption of contaminated humanitarian relief food: Uganda, March-April 2019. BMC Public Health. 2022 Mar 30;22(1):623. doi: 10.1186/s12889-022-12854-1. PMID: 35354446; PMCID: PMC8969350.

Sara, A. Review on Pharmacology of Atropine, Clinical Use and Toxicity. Biomedical and Pharmacology Journal, 15(2) June 2022. DOI: http://dx.doi.org/10.13005/bpj/2408

Kohnen-Johannsen, K.L., Kayser, O. Tropane Alkaloids: Chemistry, Pharmacology, Biosynthesis and Production. Molecules. 2019 Feb; 24(4): 796. doi: 10.3390/molecules24040796 PMCID: PMC6412926 PMID: 30813289

Alizadeh A, Moshiri M, Alizadeh J, Balali-Mood M. Black henbane and its toxicity - a descriptive review. Avicenna J Phytomed. 2014 Sep;4(5):297-311. PMID: 25386392; PMCID: PMC4224707.

---

Arbia F, Ayari-Gribaa O, Souilem F, Chiboub W, Zardi-Berguaoui A, Jannet HB, Ascrizzi R, Flamini G, Harzallah-Skhiri F. Profiles of the Essential Oils and Headspace Analysis of Volatiles from Mandragora autumnalis Growing Wild in Tunisia. Chem Biodivers. 2019 Oct;16(10):e1900345. doi: 10.1002/cbdv.201900345. Epub 2019 Sep 11. PMID: 31390142.

Srinivasan P, Smolke CD. Biosynthesis of medicinal tropane alkaloids in yeast. Nature. 2020 Sep;585(7826):614-619. doi: 10.1038/s41586-020-2650-9. Epub 2020 Sep 2. PMID: 32879484; PMCID: PMC7529995.

DeKorne, J. (2011). Psychedelic Shamanism: The Cultivation, Preparation, and Shamanic Use of PsychoTropic Plants (Kindle ed.). Amazon.

Brusselll, D. E. (2004). Medicinal Plants of Mt. Pelion, Greece. *Economic Botany, 58*, S174–S202. http://www.jstor.org/stable/4256917

Wogan, P. (2003). Magical Writing in Salasaca: Literacy and Power in Highland Ecuador (Kindle ed.). Amazon.

Muraresku, B.C. (2020). Immortality key: the secret history of the religion with no name (Kindle ed.). Amazon.

Ustinova, Y. (2017) Divine mania: alteration of consciousness in ancient Greece (Kindle ed.). Amazon.

Nixey, C. (2017). The Darkening age: the christian destruction of the classical world (Kindle ed.). Amazon.

Bohak, Gideon. A History of Jewish Magic. Amazon Kindle Edition. (2008).

Brown, Peter J. *Understanding and Applying Medical Anthropology* (1998) Mayfield Publishing Company.

Dafni, Amots., Blanche, C., Khatib, S.A., Petanidou,T., Aytac, B., Pacini, E., Kohazorva, E., Geva-Kleinberger, A., Shahvar, S., Dajic, Z., Klug, H.W., Benitez, G. In search of traces of the mandrake myth: the historical, and ethnobotanical roots of its vernacular names. (2021). *Journal of Ethnobiology and Ethnomedicine. 17*(68).

Maravi, P., Atropine eye-drop-induced acute delirium: a case report. 2020 National Institutes of Health (NIH) (.gov) https://www.ncbi.nlm.gov article PMC7223267

Plotkin, Mark J. (1993). The Shaman's Apprentice (Kindle ed.). Amazon.

Wade, Nicholas.,"Scanning an Ancient Biblical Text That Humans Fear to Open" NYT 05JAN2018 Online edition

Berlin, A., Brettler, M.Z. (2003). The Jewish Study Bible (Kindle ed.). Amazon.

Salavert, A., Zazzo, A., Martin, L. *et al.* Direct dating reveals the early history of opium poppy in western Europe. *Sci Rep* 10, 20263 (2020). https://doi.org/10.1038/s41598-020-76924-3

Braidwood, Robert J., Braidwood, Jonathan D. Sauer, Hans Helbaek, Paul C. Mangelsdorf., Cutler, Hugh C., Coon, Carleton S., Lenton, Ralph., Steward, Julian., Oppenheim, Leo

A. Did Man Once Live by Beer Alone? (1953). *American Anthropologist, 55.* pp. 515-526.

Baur, Susan Wise. "History of the Ancient World: From the Earliest Accounts to the Fall of Rome." (2001). Amazon Kindle Edition.

Doce, E. Guera,. Herrada, C. Rihuete,. Mico, R., Risch, R., Lull, V., Niemeyer, H. M. Direct Evidence of the Use of Multiple Drugs in Bronze Age Menorca (Western Mediterranean) From Human Hair Analysis.

Laumer, I. B., Rahman, A., Ramaeti, T., Azhari, U., Sri Suci, H., Atmoko, U., Schuppli, C. "Active self-treatment of a facial wound with a biologically active plant by a male Sumatran orangutan." (2024). *Scientific Reports. 14,* 8932.

Liu, Li., Wang, J., Rosenberg, D., Zhao, H., Lengyel, G., Nadel, D. Fermented beverage and food storage in 13,000y-old stone mortars at Raqefet Cave, Israel: Investigating Natufian ritual feasting. (2018). *Journal of Archaeological Science. 21,* 783-793.

Liu, Li., Wang, J., Sun, H., Chen, X. Serving red rice beer to the ancestors ca. 9000 years ago at Xiaohuangshan early Neolithic site in south China. (2023).

Pryor, Francis. "Britain BC: Life in Britain and Ireland Before the Romans." (2003). Amazon Kindle Edition.

Jacobs, Andrew., "Tripping in the Bronze Age" 19OCT2023. New York Times. Online edition

Yuval, Noah Harari. "Sapiens a Brief History of Humankind." (2011). Amazon Kindle Edition.

Katz, Josh., Sanger-Katz, Margot., Elleen Sullivan. NYT 05OCT2023 "Some Key Facts About Fentanyl" Online edition.

---

## ABOUT THE AUTHOR

---

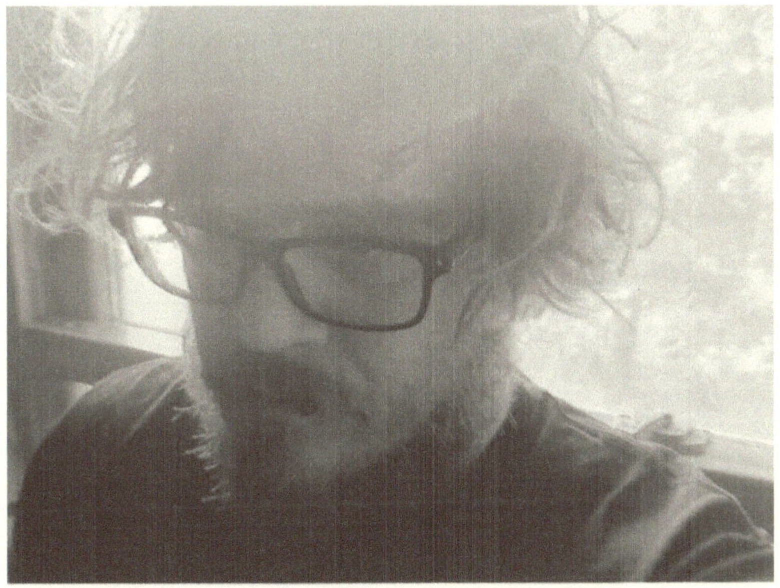

A.MICHAEL SYLM WAS born in 1983, thinks monkeys are cool and watches boxing. He has a degree from the University of Phoenix and is a father of two.

Page left black intentionally

Page left blank intentionally

Page left blank intentionally

Eisenhower Matrix consists of four quadrants: Urgent and Important, Important but Not Urgent, Urgent but Not Important, and Not Urgent and Not Important. Each quadrant represents a different category of tasks based on their urgency and importance. To apply the Eisenhower Matrix to delegation, leaders begin by creating a simple grid and categorizing tasks accordingly. By systematically assessing tasks through the lens of urgency and importance, leaders can determine the most appropriate course of action for delegation. This structured approach empowers leaders to prioritize tasks effectively and delegate responsibilities to the appropriate individuals, optimizing productivity and driving organizational success.

## Quadrant 1: Urgent and Important Tasks

Tasks in Quadrant 1 demand immediate attention and are critical to achieving organizational goals. These tasks often arise unexpectedly and require decisive action to prevent negative consequences. Examples of tasks in Quadrant 1 include addressing customer emergencies, resolving critical issues, or meeting urgent deadlines. When delegating tasks in Quadrant 1, leaders must prioritize those that align with team members' strengths and capabilities, ensuring prompt and effective resolution while maintaining a sense of urgency. By empowering team members to take ownership of urgent and important tasks, leaders can mitigate risks, capitalize on opportunities, and drive positive outcomes for the organization.

## Quadrant 2: Important but Not Urgent Tasks

In Quadrant 2, we encounter tasks that contribute to long-term success but lack immediate time sensitivity. While these tasks may not demand immediate attention, neglecting them can lead to missed opportunities or preventable crises. Examples of tasks in Quadrant 2 include strategic planning, professional development, and relationship-building initiatives.

Effective delegation in Quadrant 2 involves proactively assigning tasks to team members based on their expertise and availability. By prioritizing tasks that align with organizational goals and objectives, leaders can foster a culture of foresight and strategic planning within the organization. Delegating tasks in Quadrant 2 empowers team members to contribute meaningfully to the organization's long-term success while freeing up leaders' time to focus on high-impact activities.

## Quadrant 3: Urgent but Not Important Tasks

Quadrant 3 encompasses tasks that appear urgent but do not significantly contribute to overarching goals or priorities. These tasks often arise from distractions or minor issues that divert attention from more critical objectives. Examples of tasks in Quadrant 3 include responding to non-urgent emails, attending unnecessary meetings, or handling administrative tasks. When delegating tasks in Quadrant 3, leaders should assess their relevance and impact on organizational outcomes. Delegating or minimizing tasks in Quadrant 3 allows leaders to allocate resources effectively and focus on higher-impact activities that align with strategic objectives. By empowering team members to handle non-urgent but essential tasks, leaders can optimize productivity and drive organizational success.

## Quadrant 4: Not Urgent and Not Important Tasks

Tasks in Quadrant 4 are neither urgent nor important and typically represent time-wasting activities or distractions. These tasks consume valuable time and resources without contributing to organizational goals or personal growth. Examples of tasks in Quadrant 4 include browsing social media, attending to trivial matters, or engaging in unproductive activities. Leaders must identify and eliminate or delegate tasks in Quadrant 4 to optimize productivity and maintain focus on tasks that align with strategic objectives. By setting boundaries, managing distractions effectively, and delegating non-essential tasks, leaders can create a culture of efficiency and effectiveness within the organization.

## Tips for Effective Delegation Using the Eisenhower Matrix

To maximize the effectiveness of delegation using the Eisenhower Matrix, consider the following tips and best practices:

- Communicate task priorities and expectations clearly to team members, aligning delegation efforts with organizational goals and objectives.

- Regularly review and reassess tasks using the Eisenhower Matrix to adapt to changing priorities and emerging opportunities.

- Provide ongoing support and guidance to team members, fostering a culture of accountability and collaboration in delegation practices. By incorporating these tips into their delegation approach, leaders can harness the full potential of the Eisenhower Matrix and achieve greater effectiveness in driving organizational success.

## Conclusion

In this chapter, the exploration of delegation highlighted the critical role it played in effective leadership and organizational success. By delving into the challenges and pitfalls associated with delegation, as well as strategies for overcoming them, the chapter provided valuable insights for leaders striving to cultivate a culture of trust, empowerment, and collaboration within their teams.

We began by examining the consequences of waiting too late to delegate, emphasizing the risks of shouldering an unsustainable workload and inhibiting both personal and organizational growth. It underscored the importance of proactive delegation, advocating for a shift in mindset that viewed delegation as a strategic decision enabling long-term sustainability and growth.

Next, the discussion turned to the dangers of over-delegating, highlighting the risks of overwhelming team members, eroding cohesion, and damaging the leader's reputation and credibility. The chapter emphasized the need for a thoughtful and strategic approach to delegation that considered the individual strengths, skills, and capacity of team members, fostering a culture of trust, accountability, and empowerment.

Finally, we explored the detrimental effects of micromanagement, emphasizing its impact on trust, morale, creativity, and productivity within the team. It advocated for a more hands-off leadership approach that empowered team members to take ownership of their work, make decisions independently, and contribute meaningfully to the organization's success.

# Chapter Five

# Embrace Autonomy

When it comes to effective delegation, autonomy emerges as a cornerstone principle that holds the potential to transform workplaces and drive organizational success. Leaders encounter a multitude of challenges that can either facilitate or hinder the cultivation of autonomy within their teams.

Amid the variety of daily demands and pressures, leaders often grapple with striking the delicate balance between providing guidance and fostering autonomy. Waiting too late to embrace autonomy, succumbing to micromanagement, or failing to provide adequate resources and support can all pose significant hurdles in the pursuit of a more empowered and productive workforce.

In this chapter, we delve into the critical importance of embracing autonomy within organizations. We explore the multifaceted benefits of autonomy, ranging from increased employee engagement and job satisfaction to enhanced innovation and organizational agility. By uncovering the strategies for empowering employees, creating a culture that values autonomy, and overcoming common challenges associated with autonomy implementation, you will be equipped with the tools and insights needed to establish a more autonomous and impactful workplace.

## Understanding Autonomy

## Autonomy in the Workplace

Autonomy in the workplace is a fundamental concept that empowers employees to make decisions and take actions independently within their designated roles and responsibilities. It involves granting individuals the freedom to exercise judgment, utilize their expertise, and choose the most suitable approach to accomplish tasks. By providing autonomy, organizations acknowledge the capabilities and insights of their employees, fostering a culture of trust and empowerment. This autonomy extends beyond merely completing assigned tasks; it encompasses the authority to innovate, solve problems creatively, and contribute proactively to the organization's objectives.

Autonomy allows employees to tailor their work methods to suit their strengths and preferences, leading to increased job satisfaction and intrinsic motivation. When individuals feel trusted and valued for their contributions, they are more likely to exhibit higher levels of engagement and commitment to their work.

Moreover, autonomy encourages continuous learning and development, as employees are encouraged to explore new ideas and approaches without fear of reprisal. So defining autonomy in the workplace sets the stage for a dynamic and adaptable organizational culture where employees feel empowered to take ownership of their work and contribute to the organization's success.

## Distinguish Autonomy from Micromanagement

It's essential to distinguish autonomy from micromanagement, as they represent opposing management styles with vastly different implications for employee well-being and organizational performance. While autonomy emphasizes trust, empowerment, and delegation of authority, micromanagement involves excessive control, scrutiny, and intervention in employees' day-to-day activities. Micromanagers often exhibit a lack of trust in their employees' abilities, resulting in a stifling work environment characterized by constant supervision and scrutiny.

Unlike autonomy, which encourages employees to take initiative and exercise independent judgment, micromanagement fosters dependency and erodes confidence. Employees subjected to micromanagement may feel demotivated, disengaged, and undervalued, as their contributions are frequently questioned or overridden by their managers. Moreover, micromanagement can impede workflow efficiency, as employees may become hesitant to make decisions or take risks for fear of reprisal or criticism. Recognizing the signs of micromanagement is crucial for managers seeking to cultivate a positive work environment that promotes autonomy and fosters employee growth and development.

# The Importance of Autonomy

## Improving Employee Engagement and Motivation

Autonomy plays a pivotal role in enhancing employee engagement and motivation within the workplace. When employees are granted autonomy, they feel a sense of ownership and responsibility for their work, leading to greater investment in achieving organizational goals. By giving employees the freedom to make decisions and pursue tasks in their own way, managers demonstrate trust and respect for their capabilities, which in turn ensures a positive psychological contract between the employer and the employee. This sense of ownership and trust cultivates a more engaging work environment where employees feel valued and empowered to contribute their best efforts.

Moreover, autonomy aligns with the principles of intrinsic motivation, as individuals are driven by their internal desire for autonomy, mastery, and purpose. When employees have autonomy over their work, they are more likely to experience intrinsic rewards such as satisfaction, fulfillment, and personal growth. This intrinsic motivation leads t

## Enhancing Job Satisfaction and Retention

Autonomy significantly impacts job satisfaction and retention by providing employees with a greater sense of control and flexibility in their work. When employees have autonomy over how they approach their tasks and make decisions, they experience a greater sense of job satisfaction and fulfillment. This satisfaction stems from the alignment between their work preferences and the autonomy granted to them, leading to a stronger sense of purpose and meaning in their roles. Additionally, autonomy allows employees to better balance their work and personal lives, reducing stress and burnout and increasing overall job satisfaction.

Furthermore, autonomy is closely linked to employee retention, as individuals are more likely to stay with organizations that provide them with autonomy and opportunities for growth. Employees who feel empowered to take ownership of their work and make meaningful contributions are less likely to seek opportunities elsewhere. By investing in autonomy, organizations can create a more stable and committed workforce, reducing turnover costs and maintaining continuity in operations.

## Promoting Creativity and Innovation

Autonomy fuels creativity and innovation within teams by providing employees with the freedom to explore new ideas, experiment with different approaches, and take calculated risks. When employees are empowered to make decisions independently and think creatively, they are more likely to generate innovative solutions to complex problems. Autonomy encourages divergent thinking and removes barriers to creativity, allowing individuals to express their unique perspectives and insights.

Moreover, autonomy promotes a culture of collaboration and knowledge sharing, where employees feel encouraged to contribute their ideas and insights without fear of judgment or criticism. By fostering an environment of trust and openness, organizations can leverage the collective intelligence of their teams to drive innovation and continuous improvement. Autonomy also encourages employees to take ownership of their ideas and projects, fostering a sense of pride and accountability for their contributions.

# Empowering Employees

## Strategies for Empowering Employees

To empower employees effectively, managers can implement various strategies that foster autonomy and responsibility. These strategies are essential for creating an environment where individuals feel valued, motivated, and empowered to contribute to the organization's success. To empower your employees:

- **Clearly Communicate Organizational Goals, Objectives, and Expectations**: Transparency regarding the organization's mission, vision, and objectives helps employees understand how their work contributes to broader goals. Clear communication fosters alignment and empowers employees to make decisions that support organizational objectives.

- **Encourage Employees to Set Their Own Goals and Objectives**: Providing opportunities for employees to define their goals cultivates a sense of ownership and investment in their work. When individuals have a stake in their objectives, they are more motivated to pursue them with enthusiasm and dedication.

- **Provide Ongoing Training and Development Opportunities**: Investing in employee development not only enhances skills and competencies but also demonstrates organizational commitment to supporting growth. Training and development empower employees to take on new challenges, expand their capabilities, and contribute more effectively to the organization.

- **Delegate Authority and Decision-Making Responsibilities to Employees**: Empowering employees with decision-making authority builds trust and confidence. Delegating tasks and responsibilities allows employees to exercise autonomy, develop leadership skills, and contribute meaningfully to the organization's success.

## Benefits of Distributing Authority and Responsibility

Distributing authority and responsibility throughout the organization yields numerous benefits, both for employees and the organization as a whole. By empowering individuals to make decisions and take initiative, organizations foster a culture of ownership, collaboration, and innovation. Benefits of distributing authority and responsibility include:

- **Fostering a Sense of Ownership and Accountability among Employees**: When employees are entrusted with authority and responsibility, they take ownership of their work and outcomes. This ownership cultivates a sense of accountability, as individuals are motivated to deliver results and uphold high standards of performance.

- **Promoting Organizational Agility and Adaptability**: Distributing authority enables organizations to decentralize decision-making processes, facilitating faster responses to changing market conditions and emerging opportunities. Empowered employees can adapt quickly to evolving circumstances, driving innovation and maintaining competitive advantage.

- **Encouraging Collaboration and Teamwork**: By distributing authority and responsibility, organizations promote collaboration and teamwork among employees. Rather than relying solely on hierarchical structures, teams collaborate across functions and departments, leveraging diverse perspectives and expertise to achieve shared objectives.

- **Harnessing the Collective Intelligence of Teams**: Empowering employees to make decisions and take initiative unlocks the full potential of teams. When individuals are encouraged to contribute their ideas and insights, organizations benefit from the collective intelligence and creativity of their workforce, driving innovation and fueling sustainable growth.

## Create a Culture of Autonomy

## Cultivate a Culture That Values Autonomy

Creating a culture of autonomy begins with creating an environment where trust, empowerment, and self-management are celebrated and encouraged. Leaders play a pivotal role in setting the tone for autonomy by demonstrating trust in their teams, empowering individuals to make decisions, and providing support rather than micromanaging. Clear communication of expectations and objectives is essential to ensure that employees understand their autonomy boundaries and feel confident in their decision-making abilities.

Organizations can also implement structures and practices that support autonomy, such as flexible work arrangements, cross-functional teams, and transparent decision-making processes. By empowering employees to choose how they work and collaborate, organizations enable individuals to leverage their unique skills and perspectives to achieve common goals. Additionally, fostering a culture of continuous learning and feedback enables employees to develop their autonomy skills and grow professionally.

Overall, cultivating a culture that values autonomy requires a commitment to trust, transparency, and empowerment at all levels of the organization. When you create an environment where individuals feel valued, respected, and supported, organizations can unleash the full potential of their teams and drive sustainable success.

## Examples of Organizations Embracing Autonomy

One example of a company embracing autonomy is Spotify. The music streaming service is known for its "Agile" organizational structure, which emphasizes autonomy and flexibility.

Spotify operates in a model they call "Squads, Tribes, Chapters, and Guilds." Squads are small, self-organizing teams focused on specific features or aspects of the product. Each squad operates with a high degree of autonomy, responsible for setting its own goals, timelines, and methods of achieving them.

Tribes are collections of squads that share a common mission, such as improving user experience or expanding the platform's reach. Tribes provide a broader context for the work of individual squads while still allowing them autonomy within their specific areas.

Chapters and Guilds provide additional support and knowledge-sharing mechanisms. Chapters consist of individuals with similar skill sets across different squads, allowing for peer mentorship and development. Guilds are informal communities of interest where employees across the organization can share knowledge and best practices.

This structure allows Spotify's employees to have a significant degree of autonomy in their work while still aligning with the company's overall mission and strategy. It fosters innovation, creativity, and a sense of ownership among employees.

Similarly, Valve Corporation, a video game developer, operates under a flat organizational structure where employees have the freedom to choose their projects and collaborate with colleagues across departments. This autonomy fosters a culture of creativity, innovation, and accountability, resulting in critically acclaimed games such as *Half-Life* and *Portal*.

## Overcome Challenges

Transitioning to a more autonomous work environment can present various challenges that organizations need to navigate effectively. One common challenge is resistance to change, as some employees may feel apprehensive about relinquishing control or adapting to new ways of working. To address this challenge, organizations can emphasize the benefits of autonomy, provide training and support to help employees develop autonomy skills, and involve them in the decision-making process to foster ownership and buy-in.

## Address Common Challenges

- **Resistance to Change**: When it comes to embracing autonomy, one of the greatest hurdles organizations face is resistance to change. This resistance often stems from the inherent fear of the unknown and the perceived loss of control over one's work. However, numerous examples showcase how organizations have successfully managed this resistance. By openly discussing the benefits of autonomy, addressing concerns, and involving employees in the decision-making process, leaders can effectively overcome resistance and foster a culture of acceptance and excitement for change.

- **Maintaining Alignment and Coordination**: Another common challenge in transitioning to autonomy is maintaining alignment and coordination across teams. Without clear structures in place, autonomy can lead to fragmentation and conflicting priorities. However, by establishing clear goals, open communication channels, and effective collaboration mechanisms, organizations can mitigate these risks. Through promoting cross-functional collaboration and leveraging technology tools, teams can stay aligned, focused, and productive even in a decentralized environment.

## Solutions and Strategies for Overcoming Challenges

- **Provide Ongoing Training and Development:**

  - Tailored Programs: Offer training programs customized to meet the specific needs of employees in an autonomous work environment. Focus on building skills such as critical thinking, adaptability, and self-management.

- Continuous Learning: Encourage a culture of continuous learning and development where employees are encouraged to seek out new opportunities for growth and skill enhancement. Provide access to online courses, workshops, and mentoring programs to support ongoing learning.

- Supportive Resources: Provide employees with resources and tools to support their autonomy, such as decision-making frameworks, time management techniques, and self-assessment tools. Offer guidance and support from mentors or coaches to help employees navigate challenges and develop their autonomy skills.

- **Implement Supportive Structures and Processes**:

  - Clear Roles and Responsibilities: Define clear roles and responsibilities for each team member to ensure accountability and alignment. Clarify decision-making authority and empower employees to take ownership of their work within their designated roles.

  - Decision-Making Frameworks: Establish transparent decision-making processes that outline how decisions are made, who is involved, and what factors are considered. Provide guidelines and support to help employees make informed decisions and navigate complex situations effectively.

  - Feedback Mechanisms: Implement feedback mechanisms to gather input from employees and stakeholders on the effectiveness of autonomy initiatives. Regularly solicit feedback through surveys, focus groups, or one-on-one meetings to identify areas for improvement and address any concerns promptly.

# The Manager's Role

## Defining the Manager's Role in Supporting Autonomy

Managers serve as linchpins in creating a culture of autonomy within their teams. They must strike a delicate balance between providing guidance and allowing employees the freedom to make decisions independently. First and foremost, managers should communicate clear expectations and objectives, outlining the boundaries within which employees can exercise autonomy. This clarity ensures that employees understand their roles and responsibilities while also feeling empowered to act autonomously within those parameters.

Moreover, managers should cultivate an environment of trust and psychological safety where employees feel comfortable taking risks and making decisions without fear of judgment or reprisal. This entails creating open channels of communication, actively soliciting input from team members, and valuing diverse perspectives. When they trust in their employees' abilities, managers not only foster a sense of ownership and accountability but also encourage innovation and creativity.

Additionally, managers play a crucial role in providing support and resources to help employees succeed in their autonomous endeavors. Whether it's offering mentorship, providing access to training and development opportunities, or removing obstacles hindering progress, managers should actively empower their teams to overcome challenges and achieve their goals. Ultimately, by embracing their role as facilitators of autonomy, managers can create a culture where employees feel valued, empowered, and motivated to perform at their best.

## Effective Coaching and Mentorship

Effective coaching and mentorship are indispensable tools for helping employees develop the autonomy skills necessary to thrive in today's dynamic work environment. Coaching involves more than just giving feedback; it's about guiding employees through self-discovery, helping them identify their strengths and areas for growth, and empowering them to set and achieve their goals. This process requires active listening, asking powerful questions, and providing constructive feedback that fosters self-awareness and personal development.

Similarly, mentorship plays a vital role in supporting autonomy development by pairing employees with seasoned professionals who can offer guidance, advice, and perspective based on their own experiences. Mentors serve as trusted advisers, sharing insights, best practices, and lessons learned to help mentees navigate challenges and seize opportunities. Through regular interactions, mentees can gain valuable knowledge and skills, build confidence, and expand their professional networks.

Moreover, effective coaching and mentorship programs require ongoing commitment and support from organizational leaders. By investing in training for managers and mentors, establishing formal mentoring programs, and providing resources for continuous learning and development, organizations can create a culture that prioritizes autonomy development.

## Conclusion

In this chapter, we've delved into the transformative power of autonomy in the workplace and its pivotal role in effective delegation. We began by defining autonomy and highlighting its distinction from micromanagement, emphasizing the importance of trust and empowerment in fostering a culture where employees can thrive.

Throughout the chapter, we explored the various benefits of autonomy, including increased employee engagement, job satisfaction, and retention. By granting individuals the freedom to make decisions and take ownership of their work, organizations can unleash creativity, innovation, and collaboration within their teams. We also discussed strategies for empowering employees, creating a culture that values autonomy, and overcoming common challenges associated with autonomy implementation.

Furthermore, we examined the critical role of managers in supporting autonomy and providing effective coaching and mentorship to help employees develop autonomy skills. Real examples of organizations illustrated how they have successfully embraced autonomy, driving positive outcomes for both employees and organizations.

In conclusion, embracing autonomy is not limited to delegating tasks; it's about fostering a culture of trust, empowerment, and accountability. As you reflect on the principles and strategies discussed in this chapter, remember that embracing autonomy is a journey—one that holds the promise of unlocking extraordinary success for your team and organization.

# Chapter Six

# Learn to Trust Others

In any collaborative endeavor, whether it's a small project team or a large organizational unit, trust is essential for fostering a positive and productive work environment. When team members trust each other, they feel confident in each other's abilities, communicate more openly and honestly, and collaborate more effectively. Trust enables individuals to delegate tasks and responsibilities with confidence, knowing that they will be completed with competence and reliability.

However, building and maintaining trust within a team is not always easy. Trust can be fragile and easily eroded by misunderstandings, conflicts, or broken commitments. In this chapter, we will examine the dynamics of trust, exploring the factors that contribute to its development and the barriers that can hinder its growth. We will also discuss practical exercises and strategies for building trust within teams, from trust-building outings to conflict-resolution techniques.

Moreover, we will explore how to overcome common trust barriers, such as addressing past trust issues, managing conflicts, fostering accountability, and continuously reassessing and reinforcing trust. By understanding these challenges and implementing proactive measures to address them, teams can cultivate a culture of trust and collaboration that empowers individuals to delegate tasks and responsibilities confidently.

# The Importance of Trust

## The Foundation of Trust

Trust is the cornerstone of effective delegation. It's the glue that holds teams together, fostering collaboration, communication, and accountability. Without trust, delegation can falter, leading to misunderstandings, missed deadlines, and decreased productivity.

Think of trust as the foundation of a sturdy house. Just as a strong foundation supports the entire structure, trust underpins every aspect of teamwork. When team members trust each other and their leader, they feel comfortable sharing ideas, expressing concerns, and taking calculated risks. This openness leads to smoother collaboration, faster problem-solving, and, ultimately, better results.

Building trust takes time and effort. It starts with getting to know your team members on a personal level—understanding their strengths, weaknesses, and communication preferences. By showing genuine interest in their well-being and professional development, you demonstrate that you value them as individuals, not just as workers.

Consistency is key to building trust. You must follow through on promises, admit mistakes, and treat everyone with fairness and respect. Trust is fragile and can be easily broken, so it's essential to maintain open lines of communication and address any issues or concerns promptly.

When trust is established within a team, it creates a positive feedback loop. Team members feel more comfortable delegating tasks to each other, knowing that they will be completed competently and on time. This confidence leads to increased autonomy and empowerment, which in turn fosters even greater trust and collaboration.

By investing in trust-building efforts and fostering a culture of openness and transparency, you lay the groundwork for a high-performing team that can tackle any challenge with confidence and cohesion.

## Getting to Know Your Team on a Personal Level

Understanding your team members on a personal level is akin to unlocking a secret recipe for success. It's not just about knowing their job titles or professional skills; it's about delving deeper to understand their passions, motivations, and aspirations. This personal connection forms the foundation of trust—the cornerstone of any strong team dynamic.

An ideal scenario is a workplace where leaders take the time to genuinely get to know each member of their team. They engage in casual conversations, inquire about hobbies and interests, and show authentic interest in their team members' lives outside of work. In this environment, barriers dissolve, and bonds strengthen as team members feel valued, respected, and understood.

Getting to know your team members personally isn't just a nicety—it's a strategic imperative. When leaders invest in building these relationships, they gain invaluable insights into their team's strengths, weaknesses, and communication styles. This deeper understanding allows leaders to tailor their approach to delegation, assigning tasks based on individual preferences and capabilities.

Moreover, personal connections foster a sense of belonging and camaraderie within the team. When team members feel seen and heard, they are more likely to go the extra mile, collaborate effectively, and support each other through challenges. This sense of unity creates a positive work culture where everyone feels valued and motivated to contribute their best work.

But building personal connections requires effort and intentionality. Leaders must carve out time for one-on-one conversations, actively listen to their team members, and demonstrate empathy and understanding. By showing genuine interest in their team's well-being, leaders lay the groundwork for trust, respect, and collaboration.

Getting to know your team members on a personal level strengthens relationships, enhances communication, and fosters a positive work environment where everyone feels valued and empowered to succeed.

## Role of Trust in Effective Delegation

Trust is the lifeblood of effective delegation, permeating every aspect of the leader-team member relationship. It serves as the glue that binds individuals together, fostering collaboration, accountability, and mutual respect. Without trust, delegation becomes a precarious balancing act, teetering on the edge of uncertainty and doubt.

At its core, trust is built on a foundation of reliability and integrity. When team members trust their leader, they have confidence that their best interests are being considered and that decisions are made with honesty and fairness. This trust empowers team members to take on new challenges, knowing that their leader has their back and will provide support and guidance as needed.

Trust also plays a crucial role in communication within the team. When trust is present, team members feel comfortable expressing their thoughts and ideas openly, knowing that they will be heard and valued. This open communication fosters collaboration and innovation, as team members freely exchange ideas and work together to find solutions to challenges.

Moreover, trust is essential for effective decision-making and problem-solving within the team. When team members trust each other, they are more likely to share information, seek feedback, and collaborate on solutions. This collective trust enables the team to make decisions quickly and confidently, even in the face of uncertainty or adversity.

Building trust within a team takes time and effort, but the benefits are well worth the investment. Leaders can foster trust by leading by example and demonstrating honesty, transparency, and integrity in their actions. They can also build trust by showing empathy and understanding toward their team members, acknowledging their contributions, and providing support and encouragement.

## How Trust Enhances Team Performance

When trust permeates throughout a team, remarkable things happen—goals are achieved more efficiently, conflicts are resolved more constructively, and individuals feel empowered to contribute their best efforts.

Trust in a team environment is about having confidence in one another's abilities, intentions, and reliability. When team members trust each other, they feel comfortable taking risks, sharing ideas, and asking for help when needed. This sense of psychological safety creates an environment where creativity can flourish and where mistakes are viewed as opportunities for growth rather than reasons for blame.

One of the most significant ways trust enhances team performance is through effective delegation. When leaders trust their team members to take on tasks and responsibilities, it not only lightens the leader's load but also empowers team members to take ownership of their work. This delegation of authority fosters a sense of autonomy and accountability, motivating individuals to perform at their best.

Moreover, trust facilitates open and honest communication within the team. Team members feel safe expressing their opinions, sharing feedback, and raising concerns without fear of judgment or reprisal. This transparency strengthens relationships, builds rapport, and fosters a culture of collaboration where everyone feels valued and heard.

Trust also plays a crucial role in problem-solving and decision-making processes. In an environment of trust, team members are more willing to engage in constructive dialogue, explore alternative perspectives, and challenge assumptions. This diversity of thought leads to more innovative solutions and better-informed decisions.

Furthermore, trust enables teams to navigate through challenges and setbacks with resilience. When faced with adversity, team members rally together, drawing upon their collective strengths and support systems. Trust fosters a sense of unity and cohesion that enables teams to weather storms and emerge stronger on the other side.

## Trust as a Pillar of Organizational Culture

Trust serves as a foundational pillar upon which the entire edifice of organizational culture stands. In modern workplaces, where change is constant and uncertainty prevails, trust is the bedrock that stabilizes and strengthens organizational culture. It permeates every aspect of the workplace, influencing employee engagement, productivity, and overall organizational performance.

At its essence, trust in organizational culture is about fostering an environment where employees feel secure, respected, and valued. It is cultivated through transparent communication, consistent actions, and genuine relationships. When trust is deeply ingrained in the culture, employees are more likely to feel a sense of belonging and loyalty to the organization.

Trust in organizational culture also manifests through leadership. Leaders who embody integrity, authenticity, and empathy inspire trust among their team members. They lead by example, demonstrating a commitment to fairness, accountability, and ethical behavior. When employees trust their leaders, they are more likely to align with the organization's vision, embrace change, and exert discretionary effort to achieve shared goals.

Furthermore, trust in organizational culture fosters collaboration and teamwork. When individuals trust each other, they are more inclined to share knowledge, leverage each other's strengths, and work toward common objectives. This collaborative spirit enhances innovation, problem-solving, and adaptability, enabling organizations to thrive in an ever-evolving marketplace.

Moreover, trust in organizational culture is a catalyst for employee engagement and satisfaction. When employees feel trusted and empowered, they are more motivated to contribute their best efforts, take initiative, and pursue continuous growth and development. This sense of autonomy and agency fosters a positive work environment where individuals can flourish and fulfill their potential.

Finally, trust in organizational culture enhances resilience and agility. In times of uncertainty or adversity, organizations built on a foundation of trust are better equipped to navigate challenges, pivot strategies, and seize opportunities. Trust fosters a culture of adaptability and resilience, where employees feel confident in their ability to overcome obstacles and drive positive change.

## Trust Exercises for Team Development

### Outings

Team outings provide opportunities for team members to bond, build rapport, and develop trust outside of the typical work environment.

These activities foster a sense of camaraderie and help team members feel more connected to each other. Here are some types of outings that can be beneficial for team development:

- **Team-Building Retreats**: Team-building retreats offer a dedicated time away from the usual work environment for team members to engage in structured activities aimed at enhancing trust, communication, and collaboration. These retreats can vary in duration and location, ranging from a one-day off-site outing to a multiday getaway. During a retreat, team members may participate in a variety of workshops, exercises, and challenges designed to strengthen teamwork and build trust. Some common activities at team-building retreats include:

  - Workshops and Seminars: Facilitated sessions focusing on topics such as effective communication, conflict resolution, and leadership development. These workshops provide opportunities for team members to learn new skills and strategies for working together more effectively.

  - Outdoor Adventure Challenges: Activities like ropes courses, zip-lining, or team-building games in natural settings encourage collaboration, problem-solving, and risk-taking. These challenges often require teams to work together to overcome obstacles and achieve shared goals, fostering trust and camaraderie.

  - Reflective Discussions and Debriefs: Scheduled times for team members to reflect on their experiences, share insights, and discuss how the lessons learned during the retreat can be applied to their work. Debriefing sessions allow teams to identify strengths, areas for improvement, and actionable steps for continued growth.

- **Outdoor Adventure Activities**: Outdoor adventure activities provide opportunities for team members to step out of their comfort zones, take on new challenges, and work together to overcome obstacles in a natural setting. These activities require teamwork, communication, and trust, as individuals rely on each other to navigate unfamiliar terrain and complete tasks successfully. Some examples of outdoor adventure activities for team building include:

  - Hiking and Backpacking: Trekking through nature trails or wilderness areas allows teams to bond while exploring new surroundings and working together to navigate trails and overcome obstacles.

  - Rock Climbing and Rappelling: Scaling rock faces or descending cliffs requires trust and collaboration between climbers and belayers. Team members must communicate effectively and support each other to ensure safety and success.

  - White-Water Rafting and Canoeing: Paddling down rivers or navigating rapids in a raft or canoe requires coordination and teamwork to steer, navigate obstacles, and stay afloat. These water-based adventures promote trust and camaraderie as teams work together to conquer the challenges of the river.

- **Social Gatherings**: Social gatherings provide opportunities for team members to relax, unwind, and connect with each other on a personal level outside of the workplace. These informal events create a relaxed atmosphere where team members can build relationships, share experiences, and foster a sense of community. Some popular social gathering ideas for team building include:

- ○ Team Lunches or Dinners: Gathering for a meal at a local restaurant or hosting a potluck lunch in the office allows team members to bond over food and conversation. Sharing a meal creates a sense of camaraderie and provides an opportunity for informal networking.

- ○ Game Nights or Movie Screenings: Organizing a game night with board games, card games, or video games encourages teamwork, competition, and laughter. Alternatively, hosting a movie night with popcorn and snacks allows team members to relax and enjoy a film together.

- ○ Sports and Recreational Activities: Participating in sports or recreational activities such as bowling, mini-golf, or karaoke promotes friendly competition and team spirit. These activities provide opportunities for team members to have fun and bond in a relaxed and informal setting.

## Exercises

In addition to team outings, specific exercises can be implemented to foster trust, collaboration, and cohesion among team members. These exercises are designed to encourage communication, problem-solving, and mutual support, ultimately strengthening the bonds within the team. These exercises can be beneficial for team development:

- **Role-Playing Scenarios**: Role-playing scenarios provide opportunities for team members to simulate real-life situations and practice their communication and interpersonal skills in a safe and controlled environment. These scenarios can be tailored to address specific challenges or conflicts that may arise in the workplace, allowing team members to explore different perspectives and develop empathy for their colleagues. Some examples of role-playing scenarios include:

- ○ Conflict Resolution: Teams can role-play common workplace conflicts, such as disagreements between team members or conflicts with clients or customers. By stepping into each other's shoes and practicing active listening and problem-solving techniques, team members can learn to resolve conflicts more effectively.

- ○ Customer Interactions: Teams can role-play interactions with customers or clients to practice delivering excellent customer service and handling difficult situations professionally. These scenarios help team members develop confidence in their communication skills and build trust with external stakeholders.

- ○ Leadership Development: Teams can role-play leadership scenarios, such as leading team meetings or coaching team members through challenges. These exercises allow team members to practice leadership skills and develop trust in their leaders' ability to guide and support them.

- **Problem-Solving Challenges**: Problem-solving challenges provide opportunities for teams to work together to tackle complex problems and find creative solutions. These challenges require collaboration, critical thinking, and decision-making skills, fostering trust and teamwork among team members as they work toward a common goal. Some examples of problem-solving challenges include:

- Escape Room Puzzles: Teams are locked in a themed room and must solve a series of puzzles and riddles to unlock the door and escape within a set time limit. These challenges require teamwork, communication, and lateral thinking to decipher clues and solve the mystery.

- Scavenger Hunts: Teams are given a list of clues or tasks to complete within a specified area, requiring them to work together to solve puzzles, navigate obstacles, and collect items. Scavenger hunts encourage collaboration, creativity, and strategic thinking as teams race against the clock to complete the challenge.

- Brainstorming Sessions: Teams are presented with a problem or opportunity and must generate ideas and solutions through brainstorming sessions. These exercises promote open communication, idea sharing, and collaboration as team members build on each other's contributions to develop innovative solutions.

- **Trust Falls and Blindfolded Activities**: Trust falls and blindfolded activities are classic team-building exercises that require trust, communication, and reliance on team members for support and guidance. These activities help to build trust and confidence among team members as they demonstrate vulnerability and rely on each other for safety and assistance. Some examples of trust falls and blindfolded activities include:

  - Trust Falls: Team members take turns falling backward into the arms of their teammates, trusting that they will be caught and supported. Trust falls encourage trust, communication, and mutual reliance as team members demonstrate their willingness to support and protect each other.

- Blindfolded Obstacle Courses: Team members navigate a series of obstacles or challenges while blindfolded, relying on verbal instructions and guidance from their teammates to navigate safely. These activities promote communication, trust, and teamwork as team members work together to overcome obstacles and reach the finish line.

- Blindfolded Drawing: Teams are given a drawing task and must work together to complete the drawing while blindfolded. One team member wears a blindfold and holds a pen or pencil, while their teammates provide verbal instructions and guidance. This activity promotes trust, communication, and collaboration as team members rely on each other to complete the task successfully.

- **Personality Assessments and Team Dynamics Workshops**: Personality assessments and team dynamics workshops are valuable tools for helping team members understand themselves and each other better, leading to improved communication, collaboration, and trust. These exercises provide insights into individual strengths, preferences, and working styles, allowing team members to appreciate and leverage their differences to achieve common goals. Here are some examples of personality assessments and team dynamics workshops:

- Myers-Briggs Type Indicator (MBTI): Team members complete the MBTI assessment to identify their personality type preferences across different dimensions, such as extraversion vs. introversion, sensing vs. intuition, thinking vs. feeling, and judging vs. perceiving. Workshops based on MBTI results help team members understand their own preferences and those of their colleagues, promoting empathy, respect, and effective communication.

- DISC Assessment: The DISC assessment categorizes individuals into four primary behavioral styles: dominance, influence, steadiness, and conscientiousness. Team members learn about their own behavioral style and how it interacts with others' styles to influence team dynamics and communication patterns. Workshops based on DISC results help teams improve collaboration, conflict resolution, and trust by fostering mutual understanding and appreciation of diverse perspectives.

- StrengthsFinder Assessment: The StrengthsFinder assessment identifies individuals' top strengths and talents, providing insights into how they can contribute most effectively to team success. Workshops based on StrengthsFinder results help team members recognize and leverage each other's strengths, leading to more effective teamwork, increased trust, and improved performance.

- **Group Discussions and Sharing Sessions**: Group discussions and sharing sessions provide opportunities for team members to engage in open and honest conversations, share their thoughts and experiences, and build connections with each other. These sessions create a supportive and inclusive environment where team members can express themselves, ask questions, and learn from each other's perspectives. Some examples of group discussions and sharing sessions include:

- Team Retrospectives: Regular meetings where team members reflect on recent projects, identify successes and challenges, and discuss lessons learned. Retrospectives encourage open communication, constructive feedback, and continuous improvement, fostering trust and accountability within the team.

- ○ Book or Article Clubs: Team members read and discuss relevant books, articles, or case studies related to their field or areas of interest. These discussions promote learning, critical thinking, and knowledge sharing, strengthening bonds and trust among team members.

- ○ Career Development Sessions: Team members share their career goals, aspirations, and challenges with each other, seeking advice, support, and mentorship from their colleagues. These sessions promote professional growth, collaboration, and trust as team members offer guidance, encouragement, and resources to help each other succeed.

# Overcome Trust Barriers

## Address Past Trust Issues

Past trust issues, whether within the team or between team members and leadership, can undermine collaboration, communication, and productivity. It's essential to address these issues openly and proactively to rebuild trust and create a positive work environment. Here are some strategies for addressing past trust issues:

- Identify the Root Causes: Start by identifying the specific incidents or behaviors that led to trust issues within the team. This may involve conducting individual or group discussions to understand each team member's perspective and experiences. By identifying the root causes of trust issues, you can develop targeted solutions to address them effectively.

- **Apologize and Take Responsibility**: If team leaders or individual team members have contributed to trust issues through their actions or behaviors, it's essential to acknowledge their mistakes, apologize sincerely, and take responsibility for their actions. Demonstrating accountability and humility can go a long way in rebuilding trust and repairing damaged relationships within the team.

- **Implement Concrete Actions**: Take concrete steps to address the underlying issues that have contributed to trust issues within the team. This may involve implementing new policies, processes, or communication strategies to prevent similar issues from arising in the future. For example, if trust issues have stemmed from a lack of transparency or information sharing, consider implementing regular updates, transparent decision-making processes, or team-building activities to foster trust and collaboration.

- **Provide Support and Resources**: Offer support and resources to help team members navigate and overcome trust issues effectively. This may include providing access to conflict-resolution training, coaching, or counseling services to help team members develop essential communication and interpersonal skills. By investing in their personal and professional development, you can empower team members to address trust issues constructively and proactively.

- **Monitor Progress and Follow Up**: Continuously monitor the progress of trust-building efforts within the team and follow up regularly to assess their effectiveness. Solicit feedback from team members to gauge their perceptions of trust and collaboration within the team and identify any ongoing challenges or areas for improvement. Adjust your approach as needed based on feedback and observations to ensure that trust issues are addressed comprehensively and sustainably over time.

## Manage Conflicts and Misunderstandings

Conflicts and misunderstandings are inevitable in any team setting, but how they are managed can significantly impact trust and collaboration. Effectively addressing conflicts and misunderstandings can prevent them from escalating and undermining trust within the team. Here are some strategies for managing conflicts and misunderstandings:

- **Promote Open Dialogue**: Encourage team members to address conflicts and misunderstandings openly and constructively. Create a culture where individuals feel empowered to express their concerns, share their perspectives, and seek resolution collaboratively. Provide opportunities for dialogue through team meetings, one-on-one discussions, or facilitated group sessions.

- **Practice Active Listening**: Ensure that all parties involved in a conflict or misunderstanding feel heard and understood by practicing active listening. Encourage team members to listen attentively to each other's viewpoints without interruption or judgment. Use techniques such as paraphrasing, summarizing, and asking clarifying questions to demonstrate understanding and empathy.

- **Seek to Understand**: Encourage team members to approach conflicts and misunderstandings with a mindset of curiosity and empathy. Encourage them to explore the underlying reasons behind each other's perspectives and behaviors to gain a deeper understanding of the situation. Foster empathy and perspective-taking to promote mutual respect and trust within the team.

- **Focus on Interests, Not Positions**: Encourage team members to focus on identifying and addressing the underlying interests and needs driving the conflict, rather than clinging to rigid positions. Help them explore win-win solutions that satisfy everyone's interests and contribute to the team's overall goals and objectives. Facilitate brainstorming and problem-solving sessions to generate creative solutions to conflicts and misunderstandings.

- **Establish Clear Communication Norms**: Set clear expectations for how communication should be conducted within the team to prevent misunderstandings and misinterpretations. Establish guidelines for respectful communication, active listening, and constructive feedback. Encourage team members to communicate openly, honestly, and transparently, and provide training or resources to help them develop effective communication skills.

- **Mediate Conflicts When Necessary**: In cases where conflicts or misunderstandings cannot be resolved independently, provide mediation or facilitation support to help facilitate constructive dialogue and find mutually acceptable solutions. Consider involving a neutral third party, such as a mediator or HR representative, to facilitate discussions and help parties find common ground.

## Instill Accountability and Responsibility

Accountability and responsibility are essential elements of a high-trust team environment. When team members hold themselves and each other accountable for their actions and commitments, trust flourishes, and collaboration thrives. Here are some strategies for enhancing accountability and responsibility within the team:

- **Set Clear Expectations**: Establish clear and achievable expectations for individual and team performance, goals, and deadlines. Ensure that team members understand their roles and responsibilities, as well as the standards of behavior and performance expected of them. Clearly communicate goals, objectives, and performance metrics to provide a framework for accountability.

- **Encourage Ownership**: Foster a culture of ownership where team members take pride in their work and are committed to achieving shared goals and objectives. Encourage autonomy and empowerment by giving team members the freedom to make decisions, take initiative, and solve problems independently. Recognize and celebrate individual and team successes to reinforce a sense of ownership and accountability.

- **Provide Support and Resources**: Support team members in meeting their commitments by providing the necessary resources, training, and support they need to succeed. Ensure that team members have access to the tools, information, and guidance they need to perform their jobs effectively. Offer coaching, mentoring, or professional development opportunities to help team members develop the skills and competencies required to fulfill their responsibilities.

- **Establish Feedback Mechanisms**: Implement regular feedback mechanisms, such as performance reviews, check-ins, or peer evaluations, to provide ongoing feedback and accountability. Encourage team members to provide feedback to each other on their performance, behavior, and contributions to the team. Use feedback as a tool for growth and improvement, rather than criticism or judgment, to promote accountability and continuous learning.

- **Address Accountability Gaps**: Address accountability gaps promptly and constructively when they arise. If team members fail to meet their commitments or perform below expectations, provide timely and specific feedback to help them course-correct and improve. Offer support and guidance to help them identify and overcome obstacles and develop strategies for success. Hold team members accountable for their actions and provide consequences for repeated or egregious violations of trust or accountability.

## Continuously Reassess and Reinforce Trust

Building and maintaining trust within a team is an ongoing process that requires regular assessment and reinforcement. By continually monitoring trust levels and taking proactive steps to reinforce trust, teams can sustain a positive and collaborative work environment. These are strategies for continuously reassessing and reinforcing trust within the team:

- **Collect Feedback**: Regularly solicit feedback from team members to gauge their perceptions of trust within the team. Use surveys, focus groups, or one-on-one conversations to gather insights into team dynamics, communication patterns, and trust levels. Ask specific questions about trust, transparency, and collaboration to identify areas for improvement and potential trust barriers.

- **Conduct Trust-Building Activities**: Organize regular team-building activities, workshops, or retreats focused on building trust and strengthening relationships within the team. These activities can include trust falls, team-building exercises, or facilitated discussions about trust and collaboration. Use these opportunities to reinforce the importance of trust, promote open communication, and address any trust issues or concerns that arise.

- **Lead with Transparency**: Foster a culture of transparency and openness by providing regular updates, sharing information openly, and involving team members in decision-making processes. Be transparent about the team's goals, objectives, and priorities, as well as any changes or challenges affecting the team. Transparency builds trust by demonstrating honesty, integrity, and respect for the team's members.

- **Celebrate Successes**: Acknowledge and celebrate the team's successes, achievements, and milestones to reinforce trust and boost morale. Recognize individual and team contributions publicly and show appreciation for their hard work and dedication. Celebrating successes fosters a sense of pride, camaraderie, and trust within the team, motivating team members to continue working collaboratively toward shared goals.

## Conclusion

As we conclude our exploration of trust within teams, it becomes evident that trust is not simply a passive component but an active catalyst for collaboration, innovation, and growth.

Throughout this chapter, we have delved into the intricate dynamics of trust, understanding its nuances and uncovering the barriers that may impede its development. We have discussed a plethora of strategies, from trust-building exercises to conflict-resolution techniques, aimed at nurturing trust within teams.

By addressing past trust issues, managing conflicts constructively, fostering accountability, and continuously reassessing and reinforcing trust, teams can create a culture where trust thrives as the bedrock of their interactions. This culture of trust not only enhances delegation processes but also fosters an environment where individuals feel empowered to take risks, share ideas, and contribute their best efforts toward common objectives.

In closing, we have to recognize trust as a fundamental principle that guides us toward effective collaboration, synergy, and shared success. When it comes to teamwork, trust holds utmost importance, shaping our collective journey toward excellence. As you move forward, prioritize building and maintaining trust within your teams, knowing that it is the cornerstone of your achievements and the key to unlocking the full potential.

# Chapter Seven

# Lead by Example

In the domain of leadership and delegation, actions speak louder than words. Leading by example isn't just a catchphrase; it's a fundamental principle that sets the tone for organizational success. As we delve into the intricacies of effective delegation, we come face to face with the profound impact of leadership behavior on team performance.

This chapter helps us illuminate the path toward mastering the art of leading by example. We'll explore the core principles that underpin this approach, dissecting the essence of working hard, embracing continual self-growth, and embodying integrity and accountability. Through these lenses, we'll uncover how leaders can inspire, motivate, and empower their teams to reach unparalleled heights of productivity and excellence.

But leading by example isn't just about individual actions; it's about fostering a culture of excellence within your organization. It's about instilling values, fostering collaboration, and cultivating a shared sense of purpose. By setting the standard and embodying the behaviors you wish to see in others, you pave the way for a harmonious and high-performing team environment.

# The Meaning of Leading by Example

## Working Hard

Working hard is the cornerstone of leading by example. As a leader, demonstrating a strong work ethic not only inspires your team members but also sets a standard of excellence within the organization. When you constantly put in the effort and show dedication to your tasks, it motivates others to do the same. Working hard involves more than just putting in long hours; it's about being proactive, focused, and committed to achieving goals. When you lead from the front and show that you're willing to roll up your sleeves and get the job done, you build trust and credibility with your team.

Furthermore, working hard instills a sense of accountability and responsibility among team members. When they see you putting in the effort, they're more likely to feel a sense of ownership over their work and strive for excellence. Additionally, working hard fosters a culture of productivity and achievement, where everyone is committed to delivering their best. Embodying the value of hard work lays the groundwork for success and inspires those around you to reach new heights.

## Continual Self-Growth

Continual self-growth is not just a goal; it's a fundamental aspect of effective leadership. It's a journey of self-discovery and improvement that requires a commitment to learning and development. Central to this journey is the willingness to accept feedback from various sources, whether it be peers, subordinates, or superiors. Feedback serves as a mirror, reflecting our strengths and weaknesses, and provides invaluable insights into areas for improvement. Effective leaders understand the importance of feedback as a catalyst for growth and actively seek it out, demonstrating humility and openness to constructive criticism.

Moreover, accepting feedback isn't enough; true growth comes from implementing changes based on the feedback received. This requires a willingness to step out of one's comfort zone and embrace new approaches or perspectives. Whether it's refining leadership styles, honing communication skills, or acquiring new knowledge, effective leaders are proactive in their pursuit of self-improvement. When they continually evolve and adapt to new challenges, leaders set a powerful example for their team members, inspiring them to embark on their own journeys of growth and development.

## Integrity and Admitting When Wrong

Integrity is the cornerstone of effective leadership. It encompasses honesty, transparency, and ethical behavior in all aspects of decision-making and interactions. At the heart of integrity lies the willingness to admit when one is wrong. It takes humility and courage to acknowledge mistakes and take responsibility for them. Leaders who demonstrate integrity earn the trust and respect of their team members, as they lead by example, showing that they are accountable for their actions.

Admitting when wrong is not a sign of weakness but rather a display of strength and character. It fosters an environment of honesty and openness where team members feel valued and respected. When leaders take ownership of their mistakes, it creates a sense of psychological safety within the team, enabling individuals to speak up without fear of judgment or reprisal. This, in turn, fosters a culture of collaboration and innovation where diverse perspectives are welcomed and considered.

## Challenges and Pitfalls

- **Consistency over Time**: Maintaining consistency in behavior and actions over time can be challenging. Leaders may face temptations to deviate from established principles or take shortcuts, especially when under pressure or facing difficult situations. Consistently upholding high standards of behavior requires discipline and self-awareness.

- **Navigating Organizational Dynamics**: Leaders must navigate the complexities of organizational dynamics and interpersonal relationships. Resistance or pushback from team members who are resistant to change or accustomed to different leadership styles may arise. Managing conflicts and fostering a positive team culture requires tact, empathy, and effective communication skills.

- **Balancing Priorities**: Finding the right balance between providing support and autonomy, being approachable yet maintaining authority, can be a delicate balancing act for leaders. Failure to strike this balance can lead to feelings of resentment or disengagement among team members.

- **Maintaining Well-Being and Resilience**: The pressure to perform, combined with long hours and high expectations, can take a toll on leaders' mental and emotional health. Prioritizing self-care and seeking support when needed is essential to avoid burnout and maintain effectiveness.

- **Failure to Address Blind Spots**: One significant pitfall is the failure to recognize and address one's own blind spots or areas for improvement. Leaders who are unwilling to acknowledge their limitations or vulnerabilities risk alienating team members and undermining trust and credibility.

In navigating these challenges and pitfalls, leaders who remain committed to leading by example can inspire their teams to achieve greatness. By addressing these obstacles head-on, leaders cultivate a culture of accountability, resilience, and growth within their organizations.

## Benefits of Assigning Tasks and Being Organized

## Increased Efficiency

Assigning tasks and being organized can significantly enhance efficiency within a team or organization. When tasks are clearly delegated and organized, team members have a clear understanding of their responsibilities and deadlines. This clarity minimizes confusion and overlap, allowing individuals to focus on their assigned tasks without wasting time on unnecessary coordination or guesswork. Moreover, efficient task assignment ensures that resources are utilized optimally, maximizing productivity and output.

Furthermore, being organized facilitates smooth workflow and prevents bottlenecks or delays in project execution. With a well-defined structure in place, team members can easily track progress, identify potential issues, and make timely adjustments as needed. This proactive approach to task management ensures that projects stay on schedule and are completed with minimal disruptions, ultimately leading to higher levels of efficiency and achievement.

## Empowerment and Growth

Assigning tasks empowers team members by providing them with clear roles and responsibilities, as well as the autonomy to make decisions within their designated areas. This empowerment fosters a sense of ownership and accountability, motivating individuals to take initiative and contribute their best efforts toward achieving shared goals. When team members feel trusted and empowered, they are more likely to demonstrate high levels of engagement, creativity, and problem-solving skills.

Moreover, task assignment serves as a vehicle for personal and professional growth. By delegating tasks that align with team members' strengths and interests, leaders provide opportunities for skill development and career advancement. As individuals take on new challenges and expand their capabilities, they gain valuable experience and confidence, paving the way for future success.

Additionally, empowerment and growth go hand in hand with a supportive organizational culture that values learning and development. By fostering an environment where individuals are encouraged to take ownership of their work and pursue continuous improvement, leaders lay the foundation for long-term success and fulfillment for both individuals and the organization as a whole.

## Better Time Management

Effective task assignment and organization contribute to better time management within a team or organization. By clearly defining tasks, deadlines, and priorities, leaders enable team members to allocate their time and resources more efficiently. This clarity reduces procrastination and indecision, allowing individuals to focus their efforts on tasks that contribute most to the overall objectives.

Furthermore, being organized facilitates effective time allocation and resource planning. With a clear understanding of project timelines and resource requirements, leaders can allocate resources strategically, ensuring that tasks are completed on time and within budget. Additionally, effective organization minimizes the risk of overcommitment or burnout, as individuals can better balance their workload and prioritize tasks based on importance and urgency.

## Enhanced Collaboration

Clear task assignment and organization promote enhanced collaboration among team members. When responsibilities are clearly defined and communicated, it fosters a sense of teamwork and shared accountability.

Team members understand how their individual contributions fit into the broader context of the project or initiative, allowing them to collaborate more effectively toward common goals.

An organized workflow also facilitates communication and coordination between team members, reducing the likelihood of misunderstandings or conflicts. When they promote a culture of collaboration and cooperation, leaders can harness the collective expertise and creativity of their team members to solve problems, generate innovative ideas, and drive organizational success.

## Reduced Stress and Burnout

Effective task assignment and organization can help reduce stress and prevent burnout among team members. When roles and responsibilities are clearly defined, it minimizes uncertainty and ambiguity, alleviating the mental burden associated with unclear expectations.

Additionally, an organized workflow ensures that tasks are distributed evenly and that team members are not overwhelmed by an excessive workload. A balanced approach to task management and workload distribution allows leaders to create a supportive work environment where individuals feel valued and respected. This, in turn, leads to higher levels of job satisfaction, improved morale, and reduced turnover rates within the organization.

## Improving Your Organization and Delegation Process

## Clarify Expectations

In the realm of effective organization and delegation, clarity of expectations stands as a cornerstone. It's not merely about assigning tasks but ensuring that everyone understands the objectives, requirements, and desired outcomes. Picture a scenario where each team member knows precisely what is expected of them, like a conductor leading an orchestra with precision. With clear expectations, there's less room for misunderstandings or confusion, resulting in smoother project execution and higher-quality outcomes.

Also, clear expectations empower team members. When individuals have a crystal clear understanding of their roles and responsibilities, they feel a sense of ownership over their work. This ownership drives motivation and commitment, as team members strive to meet and exceed expectations. Clarity in expectations also allows team members to prioritize tasks effectively, ensuring that time and resources are allocated efficiently toward achieving organizational goals.

## Match Tasks to Skills

Effective delegation involves more than just assigning tasks; it's about matching tasks to the skills and capabilities of team members. Imagine a puzzle where each piece fits perfectly into place, contributing to the completion of the picture. Similarly, when tasks align with the strengths and expertise of team members, it maximizes productivity and efficiency.

Matching tasks to skills not only optimizes performance but also fosters a sense of fulfillment and engagement among team members. When individuals are assigned tasks that align with their interests and abilities, they feel valued and motivated to excel. Moreover, it provides opportunities for skill development and growth, as team members are challenged to expand their capabilities and take on new responsibilities.

Furthermore, strategic task assignment promotes collaboration and synergy within the team. When each member is working on tasks that complement their skills, it enhances overall team performance and drives organizational success.

## Provide Resources and Support

Supporting team members with the necessary resources and support is essential for effective delegation and organizational success. Imagine a gardener nurturing a garden with care, providing the right soil, water, and sunlight for each plant to thrive. Similarly, leaders should provide their team members with the tools, training, and guidance needed to succeed.

This support goes beyond tangible resources; it includes mentorship, coaching, and emotional support as well. When team members feel supported by their leaders, they are more confident in taking on new challenges and overcoming obstacles. Moreover, it fosters a culture of trust and collaboration, where team members feel comfortable seeking help and sharing ideas.

Additionally, providing resources and support demonstrates leadership's commitment to the well-being and growth of their team members. It builds loyalty and engagement, as team members feel valued and appreciated for their contributions.

## Encourage Feedback

Encouraging feedback is crucial for fostering a culture of continuous improvement and innovation within the team. It's about creating an environment where everyone feels valued and empowered to share their thoughts and ideas openly. Imagine a brainstorming session where each idea is welcomed and explored with curiosity and enthusiasm. Similarly, leaders should create opportunities for feedback, whether through regular check-ins, team meetings, or anonymous surveys.

Feedback serves as a catalyst for growth and development, providing valuable insights into what's working well and where improvements can be made. When team members feel heard and respected, they are more likely to take ownership of their work and contribute their best efforts. Moreover, feedback fosters trust and transparency within the team, strengthening relationships and collaboration.

Leaders should also lead by example by soliciting feedback on their own performance and being open to constructive criticism. This creates a culture of mutual respect and accountability, where everyone is committed to continuous learning and improvement.

## Cultural Considerations

Consideration of cultural factors is essential for effective organization and delegation, particularly in diverse teams or international settings. Cultural differences in communication styles, work habits, and decision-making processes can impact how tasks are assigned and executed. Leaders should be mindful of these cultural nuances and adapt their approach accordingly to ensure that all team members feel valued and included.

One of the key aspects of cultural consideration is communication. Different cultures may have varying norms regarding directness, hierarchy, and conflict resolution. Leaders should tailor their communication style to accommodate these cultural differences, ensuring that messages are understood and well-received by all team members.

Moreover, leaders should foster an inclusive work environment where diversity is celebrated and respected. This involves promoting cultural awareness and sensitivity among team members and addressing any biases or prejudices that may arise. By embracing cultural diversity, leaders can harness the unique perspectives and talents of their team members, driving innovation and creativity within the organization.

Furthermore, cultural consideration extends to decision-making processes and team dynamics. Leaders should be mindful of cultural differences in how decisions are made and ensure that all voices are heard and respected. So by promoting inclusivity and equity in decision-making, leaders can create a cohesive and collaborative team culture where everyone feels valued and empowered to contribute their best.

## Emotional Intelligence

Emotional intelligence is a critical component of effective leadership, encompassing the ability to recognize, understand, and manage both one's own emotions and those of others. Leaders with high emotional intelligence are adept at navigating complex interpersonal dynamics, inspiring trust and collaboration, and fostering a positive organizational culture. In this section, we will explore the various facets of emotional intelligence and how they contribute to effective organization and delegation.

## Role of Empathy

Empathy lies at the heart of emotional intelligence, enabling leaders to understand and connect with the experiences and emotions of others. Empathetic leaders listen actively, seek to understand different perspectives, and demonstrate compassion and concern for their team members. By putting themselves in others' shoes, leaders can build stronger relationships, resolve conflicts more effectively, and motivate team members to achieve common goals. Moreover, empathy fosters a sense of psychological safety within the team, where individuals feel valued and supported, leading to higher levels of engagement and job satisfaction.

## Importance of Self-Awareness

Self-awareness is another crucial aspect of emotional intelligence, involving an honest and accurate understanding of one's own emotions, strengths, weaknesses, and impact on others. Self-aware leaders recognize their triggers, biases, and patterns of behavior, allowing them to manage their emotions more effectively and make informed decisions. Additionally, self-awareness enables leaders to seek feedback, reflect on their actions, and continuously strive for personal and professional growth. Cultivating self-awareness helps leaders to set a positive example for their team members and encourages them to embrace introspection and self-improvement.

## Effective Communication

Effective communication is a key skill that stems from emotional intelligence, allowing leaders to convey their thoughts, ideas, and expectations clearly and empathetically. Emotionally intelligent leaders are attuned to nonverbal cues, such as body language and tone of voice, and adapt their communication style to resonate with their audience. They communicate with authenticity, transparency, and empathy, fostering trust and credibility among team members. Moreover, emotionally intelligent leaders are skilled listeners, creating space for open dialogue and collaboration where every voice is valued and respected. By prioritizing effective communication, leaders enhance team cohesion, alignment, and productivity, ultimately driving organizational success.

## Resilience and Adaptability

Resilience and adaptability are essential qualities that are nurtured by emotional intelligence. Resilient leaders remain calm and composed in the face of adversity, bouncing back from setbacks and maintaining a positive outlook. They view challenges as opportunities for growth and learning, rather than insurmountable obstacles. Additionally, emotionally intelligent leaders are adaptable and able to flexibly adjust their strategies and approaches in response to changing circumstances or feedback.

This adaptability enables leaders to navigate uncertainty and ambiguity with confidence, inspiring resilience and agility within their teams. By modeling resilience and adaptability, leaders promote a culture of innovation, resilience, and continuous improvement, where individuals are empowered to overcome challenges and thrive in any environment.

## Cultivating Emotional Intelligence

Cultivating emotional intelligence is an ongoing journey that requires self-reflection, practice, and commitment. Leaders can enhance their emotional intelligence through mindfulness practices, such as meditation and journaling, which promote self-awareness and emotional regulation. Additionally, seeking feedback from trusted mentors or coaches can provide valuable insights into blind spots and areas for improvement. Developing empathy and effective communication skills can be furthered through active listening, empathy exercises, and role-playing scenarios. Prioritizing the development of emotional intelligence allows leaders to create a supportive and inclusive work environment where individuals feel valued, empowered, and inspired to achieve their full potential.

## Long-Term Impact

Understanding the long-term impact of effective organization and delegation goes beyond immediate results; it encompasses the broader implications for organizational culture, employee morale, and overall success.

## Influence on Organizational Culture

Effective organization and delegation practices have a profound impact on organizational culture, shaping the values, norms, and behaviors that define the workplace environment. When leaders prioritize clarity, transparency, and accountability in task assignment and workflow management, it sets a positive tone for the entire organization. Clear expectations and open communication foster trust and collaboration among team members, creating a culture of transparency and mutual respect. Moreover, when employees feel empowered to take ownership of their work and contribute meaningfully to the organization's goals, it fosters a sense of pride and engagement. A healthy organizational culture built on effective organization and delegation practices promotes innovation, creativity, and resilience, driving long-term success.

## Employee Morale

Effective organization and delegation directly impact employee morale and job satisfaction. When tasks are assigned strategically and resources are allocated efficiently, it reduces stress and burnout among team members. Clear expectations and support from leadership contribute to a positive work environment where individuals feel valued, motivated, and engaged. Moreover, when employees are empowered to make decisions and take ownership of their work, it fosters a sense of autonomy and fulfillment. High morale leads to higher levels of productivity, creativity, and loyalty, as employees are more likely to go above and beyond to support organizational goals.

## Overall Success

The long-term success of an organization hinges on its ability to adapt, innovate, and thrive in a dynamic and competitive environment. Effective organization and delegation lay the foundation for sustainable growth and resilience by optimizing resources, maximizing productivity, and fostering a culture of continuous improvement. When tasks are assigned strategically and aligned with organizational goals, it ensures that efforts are focused on high-priority initiatives that drive value and innovation. Moreover, when employees are empowered to take ownership of their work and collaborate effectively, it unleashes the full potential of the team, leading to greater creativity, innovation, and problem-solving. So, organizations that prioritize effective organization and delegation practices are better positioned to navigate challenges, seize opportunities, and achieve long-term success in today's rapidly evolving business landscape.

## Conclusion

Throughout this chapter, we've delved into the essence of what it means to embody this principle and the profound impact it can have on team dynamics and organizational success.

From the foundational pillars of working hard and embracing continual self-growth to the cornerstone of integrity and accountability, we've explored the key qualities that define exemplary leadership. By setting a strong example and fostering a culture of excellence, leaders can ignite a spark within their teams, driving them toward unprecedented levels of productivity and achievement.

Moreover, we've discussed the tangible benefits of assigning tasks and maintaining organizational efficiency. By empowering team members, providing support, and clarifying expectations, leaders can unleash the full potential of their teams while simultaneously ensuring smooth workflow and optimal resource utilization.

As we conclude our journey through the foundations of leading by example and effective delegation, it's crucial to remember that leadership is not a destination but a continuous journey of growth and development. By embracing the principles outlined in this chapter and striving for excellence in every endeavor, we can cultivate environments where individuals thrive, teams flourish, and organizations excel.

So, as you navigate your leadership journey, remember the power you hold to shape the future through your actions and behaviors. Lead with purpose, integrity, and humility, and watch as your influence creates ripples of positive change far beyond what you can imagine.

# Chapter Eight

# The Art of Appreciation

The Art of Appreciation is not just a nicety; it's a strategic imperative for organizations seeking to thrive in today's competitive landscape. By fostering a culture of gratitude, leaders can unlock the full potential of their teams, driving engagement, innovation, and performance. Whether through simple acts of saying "thank you" or systematic recognition programs, every gesture of appreciation contributes to a workplace environment where individuals feel valued, motivated, and empowered to achieve their goals. As leaders embrace the art of appreciation, they not only cultivate a positive work culture but also lay the foundation for long-term success and sustainability.

In this chapter, we will delve into the transformative power of appreciation and its multifaceted impact on employee morale, motivation, and performance. From recognizing contributions to fostering motivation and providing constructive criticism, we'll explore various aspects of appreciation that leaders can leverage to create a positive work environment and drive organizational success. Through practical strategies and insights, we aim to equip leaders with the tools they need to cultivate a culture of gratitude within their organizations.

# The Power of "Thank You"

## Recognizing Contributions

In any organization, every member of the team plays a crucial role in its success. Whether it's a significant project milestone, a small but impactful contribution, or consistent dedication to the team's objectives, each effort deserves acknowledgment.

Recognizing these contributions isn't merely a formality; it's an essential aspect of effective leadership. When leaders take the time to acknowledge and appreciate the efforts of their team members, it reinforces their value within the organization. This validation not only boosts morale but also fosters a sense of belonging and commitment among employees.

Moreover, recognition cultivates a culture of appreciation within the workplace. When employees see their efforts being acknowledged and rewarded, they are more motivated to continue performing at their best. This positive reinforcement not only boosts individual performance but also strengthens team dynamics and collaboration.

## Fostering Motivation

Gratitude serves as a potent catalyst for motivation within the workplace. When employees feel genuinely appreciated for their contributions, it instills a sense of pride and purpose in their work. A simple "thank you" or acknowledgment of their efforts can have a profound impact on their morale and motivation.

Expressing gratitude fosters a positive feedback loop. As employees receive recognition for their hard work, they are more likely to feel valued and respected by their peers and leaders. This, in turn, strengthens their commitment to the organization and motivates them to continue striving for excellence.

Furthermore, a culture of gratitude encourages employees to go above and beyond in their roles. When individuals feel appreciated, they are more inclined to take initiative, solve problems creatively, and collaborate effectively with their colleagues. This proactive approach to work not only benefits individual performance but also contributes to the overall success of the organization.

# Provide Constructive Criticism

Constructive criticism is a cornerstone of personal and professional development within any organization. It's a process that involves delivering feedback in a manner that is intended to be helpful, insightful, and focused on growth rather than judgment. In this section, we explore the significance of constructive criticism and offer detailed strategies for delivering it effectively.

## Understanding the Importance of Constructive Criticism

Constructive criticism serves as a catalyst for improvement by helping individuals identify areas where they can enhance their skills and performance. Unlike destructive criticism, which focuses solely on faults and shortcomings, constructive criticism aims to provide actionable insights that facilitate learning and development.

Moreover, constructive criticism fosters a culture of openness and transparency within the organization. When feedback is delivered constructively, individuals feel valued and respected, and they are more likely to engage in self-reflection and take proactive steps to address areas for improvement.

Additionally, constructive criticism promotes accountability and responsibility. When they detect areas where improvement is needed and provide guidance on how to achieve it, leaders empower individuals to take ownership of their development and strive for excellence in their work.

## Key Principles of Constructive Criticism

- **Focus on Behavior**: When delivering constructive criticism, it's important to focus on specific behaviors or actions rather than making judgments about a person's character or personality. By pinpointing specific behaviors that need improvement, individuals can better understand what they need to change or adjust.

- **Be Specific and Objective**: Constructive criticism should be based on observable facts and evidence rather than subjective opinions or assumptions. Providing specific examples and evidence to support feedback helps individuals understand exactly what they did well and where they need to improve.

- **Offer Solutions and Guidance**: Simply pointing out problems without offering solutions is not constructive. Instead, provide actionable suggestions and guidance on how individuals can address the areas for improvement. This empowers individuals to take concrete steps toward growth and development.

- **Maintain a Positive Tone**: The manner in which feedback is delivered significantly impacts its effectiveness. Constructive criticism should be delivered in a respectful and positive manner, emphasizing the individual's strengths and potential for growth. Avoid using language that is harsh, critical, or demotivating, as this can undermine the individual's confidence and willingness to improve.

## Strategies for Delivering Constructive Criticism

- **Choose the Right Time and Place**: Select a time and place for delivering feedback where both parties can have a private and uninterrupted conversation. Avoid delivering criticism in front of others, as this can be embarrassing and counterproductive.

- **Use the "Sandwich" Approach**: Start and end the feedback conversation with positive comments or praise, sandwiching the criticism in between. This approach helps to soften the impact of the criticism and maintain the individual's self-esteem while still providing valuable feedback for improvement.

- **Ask for Input and Feedback**: Encourage open dialogue by inviting the individual to share their perspective on the feedback and how they plan to address it. Listen actively to their responses and be open to their ideas and suggestions for improvement.

- **Follow Up and Support**: Providing ongoing support and encouragement is essential for ensuring that constructive criticism leads to meaningful change. Check in with the individual regularly to see how they are progressing and offer additional guidance or support as needed. Recognize and celebrate their efforts and improvements to reinforce positive behaviors and encourage continued growth.

Providing constructive criticism is a skill that requires empathy, tact, and a genuine desire to support the growth and development of others. By adhering to key principles and employing effective strategies for delivering feedback, leaders can create a culture where individuals feel valued, empowered, and motivated to reach their full potential.

# Rewards and Recognition

## Tangible Rewards

Implementing tangible rewards is a concrete way to show appreciation for exceptional performance and dedication within the organization. While verbal recognition and expressions of gratitude are essential, tangible rewards provide a tangible symbol of appreciation that can have a lasting impact on employee morale and motivation.

Tangible rewards can take various forms, such as bonuses, promotions, or tangible gifts. These rewards serve as tangible manifestations of the organization's appreciation for the hard work and dedication of its employees. They not only provide a sense of validation for the recipient but also serve as a motivator for other team members to strive for similar recognition.

Moreover, tangible rewards can serve as powerful incentives for driving desired behaviors and outcomes within the organization. By linking rewards to specific performance metrics or milestones, leaders can motivate employees to focus their efforts on achieving key objectives and goals.

## Nonmonetary Recognition

While tangible rewards such as bonuses or promotions are valuable forms of appreciation, nonmonetary recognition holds equal importance in fostering a culture of appreciation within the organization. Nonmonetary recognition encompasses a wide range of gestures and practices aimed at acknowledging and celebrating the contributions of employees beyond financial incentives.

Nonmonetary recognition can take various forms, including verbal praise, written thank-you notes, public acknowledgment during team meetings or company-wide communications, and personalized tokens of appreciation such as certificates or plaques. These gestures may seem small, but they carry significant meaning and can have a profound impact on employee morale and motivation.

One of the key advantages of nonmonetary recognition is its inclusivity and accessibility. Unlike tangible rewards, which may be limited by budget constraints or organizational policies, nonmonetary recognition can be extended to all employees, regardless of their role or level within the organization. This inclusivity helps to foster a sense of belonging and camaraderie among team members, strengthening the fabric of the organizational culture.

Nonmonetary recognition also serves as a powerful tool for reinforcing desired behaviors and values within the organization. By publicly acknowledging and celebrating individuals who exemplify core values or go above and beyond in their roles, leaders can set positive examples for others to follow, driving cultural alignment and organizational success.

## Celebrating Milestones

Recognizing and celebrating significant milestones and achievements is a fundamental aspect of fostering a culture of appreciation within the organization. Whether it's reaching a project milestone, surpassing performance targets, or commemorating years of service, these milestones represent important moments in the journey of both individual employees and the organization as a whole.

Celebrating milestones serves as an opportunity to reflect on past achievements and recognize the collective efforts that contributed to them. It not only acknowledges the hard work and dedication of employees but also reinforces a sense of pride and accomplishment within the team.

Moreover, celebrating milestones helps to build camaraderie and strengthen team cohesion. By coming together to acknowledge and celebrate shared successes, employees develop a sense of unity and solidarity, fostering a supportive and collaborative work environment.

Furthermore, celebrating milestones can serve as a morale booster and motivator for employees. It provides a tangible reminder of the progress made and the impact of their efforts, instilling a sense of purpose and pride in their work. This, in turn, can inspire employees to continue striving for excellence and contributing to the organization's success.

## Amplifying Appreciation through Rituals and Traditions

### Establishing Rituals

Establishing rituals centered around appreciation is an effective way to institutionalize gratitude within the organizational culture. These rituals provide regular opportunities for team members to express appreciation for one another's contributions and reinforce the importance of recognition in the workplace. Here are some appreciation rituals:

- **Weekly or Monthly Shout-outs**: Dedicate time during team meetings to publicly acknowledge and thank team members for their contributions and achievements. This can be done through verbal praise or written notes, allowing team members to express appreciation for each other's efforts in a supportive and collaborative environment.

- **Peer-to-Peer Recognition Programs**: Implement programs that empower team members to recognize and celebrate each other's achievements. This could involve a peer-to-peer recognition platform where team members can nominate their

www.ingramcontent.com/pod-product-compliance
Lightning Source LLC
Chambersburg PA
CBHW030405160726
47992CB00007B/2963